Tissue Glues in Cosmetic Surgery

Tissue Glues in Cosmetic Surgery

EDITED BY

RENATO SALTZ, M.D.
Private Practice, Salt Lake City, Utah

DEAN M. TORIUMI, M.D.
Professor, Department of Otolaryngology,
University of Illinois,
Chicago, Illinois

COVER ILLUSTRATION
Arthur Baldissara ■ Margareth Baldissara

Quality Medical Publishing, Inc.
ST. LOUIS, MISSOURI
2004

Printed in Canada

This book presents current scientific information and opinion pertinent to medical professionals. It does not provide advice concerning specific diagnosis and treatment of individual cases and is not intended for use by the layperson. Medical knowledge is constantly changing. As new information becomes available, changes in treatment, procedures, equipment, and the use of drugs becomes necessary. The editors/authors/contributors and the publisher have, as far as it is possible, taken care to ensure that the information given in this text is accurate and up to date. However, readers are strongly advised to confirm that the information, especially with regard to drug usage, complies with the latest legislation and standards of practice. The authors and publisher will not be responsible for any errors or liable for actions taken as a result of information or opinions expressed in this book.

The publishers have made every effort to trace the copyright holders for borrowed material. If they have inadvertently overlooked any, they will be pleased to make the necessary arrangements at the first opportunity.

PUBLISHER Karen Berger
PROJECT MANAGER Mary Espenschied, Donna Rothenberg
ASSOCIATE EDITOR Michelle Berger
PRODUCTION Carolyn Reich, Susan Trail
COVER DESIGN Diane Beasley

Quality Medical Publishing, Inc.
11970 Borman Drive, Suite 222
St. Louis, Missouri 63146
Telephone: 1-800-348-7808
Web site: *http://www.qmp.com*

LIBRARY OF CONGRESS CATALOGING-IN-PUBLICATION DATA

Tissue glues in cosmetic surgery / edited by Renato Saltz, Dean M. Toriumi.—1st ed.
p. ; cm.
Includes bibliographical references and index.
ISBN 1-57626-174-3 (hard cover)
1. Adhesives in surgery. 2. Surgery, Plastic. [DNLM: 1. Reconstructive Surgical Procedures—methods. 2. Fibrin Tissue Adhesive—therapeutic use. 3. Tissue Adhesives—therapeutic use. WO 600 T6163 2004] I. Saltz, Renato. II. Toriumi, Dean M.
RD73.A3T55 2004
617.9′52—dc22

2003015283

TG/F/F
5 4 3 2 1

CONTRIBUTORS

Barbara J. Beal, B.S., R.N., C.P.S.N., C.N.O.R.
Clinical Coordinator, Craniofacial Surgery, Department of Plastic and Reconstructive Surgery, Providence Hospital, Southfield, Michigan

Ewaldo Bolivar de Souza Pinto, M.D.
Plastic Surgery Service, Unisanta, Santos SP, Brazil

Sandra G. Burks, B.S.N.
Associate Director, Surgical Therapeutic Advancement Center, University of Virginia, Charlottesville, Virginia

Ross A. Clevens, M.D.
Center for Facial Cosmetic Surgery, Melbourne and Merritt Island, Florida

Barry E. DiBernardo, M.D.
Chief, Department of Plastic Surgery, Mountainside Hospital, Montclair, New Jersey; Clinical Assistant Professor, Division of Plastic Surgery, University of Medicine and Dentistry of New Jersey, Newark, New Jersey

David A.F. Ellis, M.D., F.R.C.S.C.
Professor, Department of Otolaryngology, University of Toronto, Toronto, Ontario, Canada

Santiago Goni, M.D.
Formerly Fellow in Plastic Surgery, College Medecine des Hopitaux de Paris, Paris, France

Ian T. Jackson, M.D., M.D.Glasg.(Hon.), D.Sc.(Hon.), F.R.C.S.Ed., F.A.C.S., F.R.A.C.S.(Hon.), F.R.C.S.Glasg.(Hon.)
Director, Institute for Craniofacial and Reconstructive Surgery; Chief, Division of Plastic Surgery, Providence Hospital, Southfield, Michigan

Christopher P. Kelly, M.D.
Institute for Craniofacial and Reconstructive Surgery, Providence Hospital, Southfield, Michigan

Martin J. MacPhee, Ph.D.
Vice President, Clearant, Inc., Gaithersburg, Maryland

Daniel Marchac, M.D.
Professor, College Medecine des Hopitaux de Paris, Paris, France

Alan Matarasso, M.D.
Associate Clinical Professor, Department of Plastic Surgery, Albert Einstein College of Medicine, New York, New York

Alfred T. Mitchell, M.D.
Division of Plastic Surgery, The University of Medicine and Dentistry of New Jersey—New Jersey Medical School, Newark, New Jersey

Robert B. Nemerofsky, M.D.
Division of Plastic Surgery, The University of Medicine and Dentistry of New Jersey—New Jersey Medical School, Newark, New Jersey

Kevin O'Grady, B.A., B.S.
Research Specialist, Department of Otolaryngology—Head and Neck Surgery, University of Illinois at Chicago, Chicago, Illinois

Heinz Redl, Ph.D.
Professor, Ludwig Boltzmann Institute for Experimental and Clinical Traumatology in the AUVA Research Center, Vienna, Austria

Ricardo C. Ribeiro, M.D.
Chairman, Division of Plastic and Reconstructive Surgery, Santa Casa da Misericórdia do Rio de Janeiro, Rio de Janeiro, Brazil

Samieh S. Rizk, M.D.
Attending, Division of Facial Plastic Surgery, Department of Otolaryngology-Head & Neck Surgery, Manhattan Eye, Ear & Throat Hospital and Lenox Hill Hospital, New York, New York

Renato Saltz, M.D.
Private Practice, Salt Lake City, Utah

William D. Spotnitz, M.D.
Professor and Chief, Division of Thoracic and Cardiovascular Surgery, University of Florida, Gainesville, Florida; Director, The Surgical Therapeutic Advancement Center, University of Virginia, Charlottesville, Virginia

Dean M. Toriumi, M.D.
Professor, Department of Otolaryngology, University of Illinois, Chicago–College of Medicine, Chicago, Illinois

Belinda K. Wilmer, M.S.
Clearant, Inc., Gaithersburg, Maryland

To our families

Marcia, Bianca, and Felipe Saltz
and
Colleen, Hannah, and Olivia Toriumi

whose support and encouragement have inspired and sustained us.

FOREWORD

It is with considerable enthusiasm that I greet the publication of *Tissue Glues in Cosmetic Surgery*. The subject is timely and the editors, Renato Saltz, M.D. and Dean M. Toriumi, M.D. are distinguished surgeons, well versed in the subject of tissue adhesives. They have made numerous original contributions to the field through their clinical and experimental studies. Drs. Saltz and Toriumi have assembled a stellar group of world experts as contributors to this work with extensive experience using tissue adhesives for coaptation of tissue or for obtaining hemostasis. This is truly the definitive reference on tissue adhesives, and it offers a wealth of valuable information for the novice as well as the experienced surgeon.

Historically, as one looks back on the different methods used over time for the coaptation of tissues, particularly skin, we note that little has changed. Although needles and sutures have improved, sewing remains the mainstay for approximating skin. Suturing, however, by its nature, is a time-consuming and inefficient endeavor that may result in unsightly, often permanent, cross-hatchings. It is disappointing that at this stage, we have not developed a suturing machine that allows us to sew more expeditiously and in a more controlled fashion as is done for clothing. Although automatic staplers are an alternative to traditional suturing, useful for intestinal anastamoses and for setting up or fixing tissues in place prior to suturing, they are not the solution. It would be wise for surgeons at this stage to skip mechanical devices and to concentrate on tissue sealants or adhesives to coapt the different biologic tissues.

This book provides the comprehensive, clinical information that is needed by the surgeon interested in learning more about tissue glues. Both natural and synthetic glues are discussed. The natural sealants include among others, fibrin, denatured collagen, as well as albumin. Of the synthetics, cyanoacrylate glues are the most popular but their use is limited to approximating the epidermis.

Of the natural sealants, fibrin glue is the one that is used most extensively because of its ability to obtain hemostasis. Aesthetic surgery has benefited from the use of fibrin glue, particularly in the performance of endoscopic forehead lifts as well as facelifts, because spraying fibrin glue causes adherence of the overlying tissue to the underlying bed, maintaining its position and avoiding the dead space that may fill up with hematoma or seroma. Fibrin glue has also been used to approximate skin grafts, and it provides a wonderful benefit to the patient in that there are no sutures to remove, no stitch abscesses, or permanent cross-hatches. Tissue sealants or adhesives are a most welcome addition to cosmetic surgery because of the multitude of advantages they offer.

This book systematically reviews the evolution of tissue sealants, the types currently available, the decision-making process for choosing tissue sealants, and the clinical applications in cosmetic surgery. Surgeons interested in incorporating these tools into their practices will gain understanding and insight from the authors' careful review of the subject. The book is filled with practical, clinical advice on using tissue glues in different clinical situations with detailed chapters on endoscopic browlift, facelift, burns, and breast and body contouring. Step-by-step descriptions of glue preparation, timing, and application are included with each chapter to provide readers with a thoroughly consistent and understandable approach to this topic. With the information provided herein, surgeons should be able to use these products successfully in a safe and efficacious manner.

For me, tissue sealants hold significant promise. I look forward to a future time when we can abandon the suture and needle for coapting tissues and instead make use of sealants to accomplish this task. In vascular surgery the objective will be hemostasis with a natural sealant such as fibrin. In nerve coaptation, perhaps the choice will be a sealant with an added nerve growth factor. Sealants with considerable and lasting tensile strength may be used to coapt a tendon, and noninflammatory sealants will be used to approximate the subcutaneous tissue and skin. Obviously this will be a great bonus and a major advance for surgery of every type. The patient, however, will be the biggest beneficiary, benefiting from reduced morbidity and relief from the trauma of suture or staple removal. Additionally, the patient will receive the aesthetic bonus of shorter, more acceptable scars.

This book fills a real need for information on this topic. It will be of particular interest to cosmetic surgeons who seek to offer their patients the best aesthetic outcomes with the least morbidity. It should also be read by surgeons of every specialty who will gain a worthwhile understanding of tissue adhesives, their applications and benefits, and how they can be incorporated into their practices.

LUIS O. VASCONEZ, M.D.
Professor and Chief, Division of Plastic Surgery,
University of Alabama at Birmingham,
Birmingham, Alabama

PREFACE

The practice of surgery is changing, fueled in large part by innovations in technology that offer surgeons improved options and outcomes for their patients. In cosmetic surgery this translates into a wide variety of options, ranging from topical treatments to tissue fillers to more invasive surgical procedures. Traditional concepts and approaches are giving way to new less invasive operative interventions. Minimally invasive surgical techniques with smaller incisions and less dissection are transforming the practice of cosmetic surgery. Patient expectations have also been heightened with a greater premium placed on a quick recovery with minimal scarring.

Tissue glues play an important role in this changing scenario, offering the potential for reduced tissue trauma, enhanced healing, improved cosmesis, and reduced morbidity. This is particularly significant in facial cosmetic surgery where early appearance and long-term results are critical. Anything that will improve early cosmesis, allow quicker resumption of normal activities, and contribute to improved appearance over the long term is a beneficial intervention.

The search for the ideal tissue sealant has been a prime motivation for surgeons throughout the ages. The goal has been a surgical sealant and adhesive that is safe, biologically compatible, with rapid action and adequate tensile strength. Dating from the introduction of the first fibrin sealant in the 1940s, interest in the use of surgical sealants has grown steadily over time, and the number of versatile tissue adhesives and sealants available to surgeons has increased dramatically in the past 5 years.

Today, tissue glues are gaining broader acceptance in cosmetic surgery. Fibrin tissue adhesives provide surgeons with an effective means of gaining hemostasis and eliminating the use of drains in some situations. In many cosmetic procedures, large areas of tissue are elevated or dissected leaving a sizeable dead space. Fibrin tissue adhesives allow the surgeon to glue tissue together and obliterate dead space. Octyl-2-cyanoacrylate shortens operative time while providing the surgeon with an effective means of closing skin incisions without the use of sutures.

We have been using tissue glues in our practices for many years with excellent results and decided benefits in patient satisfaction. By incorporating tissue sealants in minimally invasive facial rejuvenation surgery, we have found that these adhesives contribute to hemostasis and patient comfort because they eliminate the need for drains. They also enhance the results of aesthetic facial procedures by reducing the rate of complications and other sequelae such as hematoma, seroma, bruising, and swelling. For us, tissue sealants are a valuable tool for improving the patient's surgical experience and making the postoperative course shorter and easier.

Despite the advantages that we have witnessed with tissue adhesives, we note that many surgeons have only limited experience and varied levels of success with them. Variability in the success with these products may result from inadequate understanding of the capability and effective use of these products. For this reason we have written this book with contributions from some of the world's leading experts on tissue adhesives and sealants. Our writing is based on our personal experience and that of our contributors, which has yielded consistent results with a high level of patient satisfaction. Our intent is to provide the reader with a comprehensive overview of tissue glues and guidance to maximize their application in various clinical situations. We hope this information will allow the cosmetic surgeon to improve surgical outcomes and decrease the recovery time associated with cosmetic surgery.

The book is organized into two parts. Part I provides an overview of the topic. Initial chapters focus on history, available tissue glues, present-day applications, and the clinical utility of platelet-rich plasma in facial plastic surgery. The fundamentals that guide the decision-making process are also explored in depth with specific information on how fibrin-based adhesives can be used for hemostasis and sealing, and how cyanoacrylates can be used for superficial skin closure. Particular attention is paid to safety parameters for tissue adhesives with emphasis on the use of tissue glues in cosmetic surgery.

Part II focuses on clinical applications. It begins with a description of applications for fibrin-based adhesives and cyanoacrylate adhesives in facial plastic surgery. Specific technical issues are discussed, as well as issues related to patient selection, preparation of the surgical site, applicators, setting time, effect on healing, and potential complications. Illustrative case presentations demonstrate time-tested methods of using fibrin-based adhesives and cyanoacrylate adhesives. In the remaining chapters the authors provide their personal approaches to using tissue glues for specific operations, including endoscopic browlift, short-incision face lift, breast and body contouring surgery, and burn care. Each chapter includes a detailed description of the operative approach, as well as instructions for the preparation and application of the adhesives.

The era of tissue glues in cosmetic surgery has arrived. As more novel materials and applications become available, the impact of surgical sealants on the ease and outcome of cosmetic procedures can only be expected to grow in scope and significance. We hope that this book provides the surgeon with insight into how to use these products to improve surgical outcomes.

RENATO SALTZ, M.D.
DEAN M. TORIUMI, M.D.

CONTENTS

PART I OVERVIEW

PART II APPLICATIONS

Tissue Glues in Cosmetic Surgery

PART

I

OVERVIEW

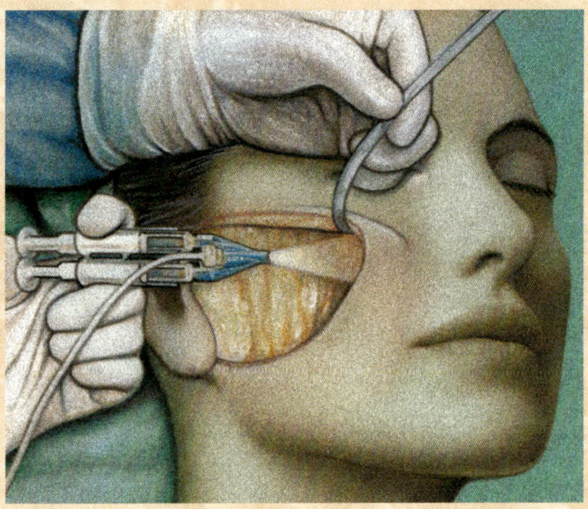

CHAPTER

1

History of Tissue Adhesives

Heinz Redl, Ph.D.

Tissue sealing has been a dream for many surgeons since time immemorial. One of the earliest attempts to use hemostats/sealants was to apply the juice of a fig tree, described in the *Iliad* "as the juice of the fig speedily maketh to grow thick the white milk that is liquid, but is quickly curdled as a man stirreth it, even so swiftly healed the furious Ares" (*Iliad* v 902-904). Evidently Homer knew that fig juice had a clotting effect on milk and by Hippocratic logic concluded it would have the same effect on blood (although the opposite is actually the case).[1]

Tissue sealing agents can be put into subcategories according to their area of efficacy:

1. To stop bleeding: hemostats
2. To close gas and liquid leaks, for example, gas leaks from lung: sealants
3. To allow the attaching of one tissue surface to another, for example, adhesives/glues: in skin transplantation

Furthermore, the tissue sealant or adhesive material should have the ability

4. To support wound healing, or at least not to interfere with this process.

Typically each of the tissue sealing agents has its forte in one of the subcategories. The fibrin sealant is the only one that fits (with limitations) into all four subcategories. In addition to being efficient for the indication needed, a tissue sealant should fulfill the criteria of

- Convenience of application
- Safety and approval for use from the authorities
- Biodegradability

On the basis of their composition, tissue sealants can be classified as natural or synthetic and further separated into a fibrin(ogen), collagen, cyanoacrylate, polyethylene glycol (PEG), albumin-glutaraldehyde, or gelatin-resorcinal-formaldehyde (GRF) product. Some historical aspects of tissue sealants have been reported previously,[2,3] and since 1996 tissue sealants have been discussed at a specialized meeting series organized by Martin J. MacPhee, William G. Spotnitz, and others.

Fibrin

Fibrin is an attractive surgical adhesive because it consists of biological components of the natural clotting cascade. In 1909 Bergel[4] demonstrated that application of fibrin powder (bovine or equine) leads to hemostasis and tissue sealing, and he postulated that fibrin powder stimulates wound healing.[4] In 1944 Tidrick and Warner[5] and Cronkite et al.[6] reported on the use of plasma fibrinogen clotted with thrombin for skin grafts.

These early attempts already suggested the basic advantages of using fibrin for wound closure, such as excellent tissue tolerance, improved wound healing, and complete in vivo resorption. Fibrin sealants were not widely accepted at that time, however, because the strength and stability of the glue were inadequate.

In 1944 E.A. Bering, Jr.,[7] reported on the preparation of fibrin foams to be used as hemostats in combination with thrombin. In 1968 a review by M. Gerendás[8] described the preparation and clinical application of (bovine) fibrin foam, fibrin powder, and fibrin films, as well as a novel slowly resorbable fibrin implant material obtained from molding a mixture of fibrin powder and a plasticizer under high pressure and temperature.

A new era in the use of fibrin sealants began in 1972, when Helene Matras (Fig. 1-1) et al.[9] successfully used a highly concentrated human plasma–derived fibrinogen solution in combination with factor XIII, thrombin, and calcium chloride to seal severed nerves in rabbit experiments.

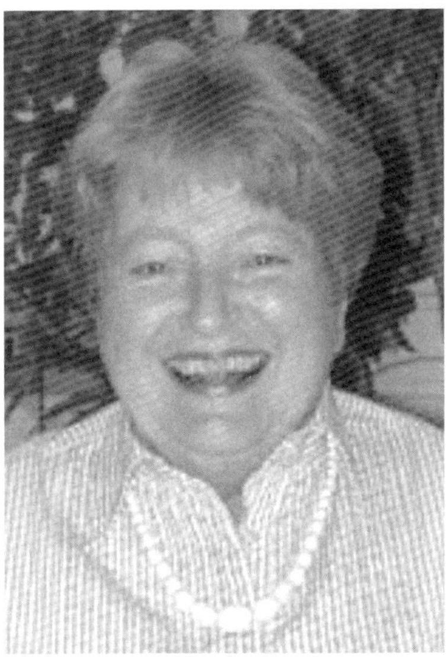

Figure 1-1 Reintroduction of tissue sealants in modern medicine in 1972 by Helene Matras, who successfully employed a fibrinogen cryoprecipitate for reuniting peripheral nerves in an animal model.[9]

Starting in 1975, Kuderna and Matras used fibrin sealant clinically for nerve anastomosis in our trauma center.[10] In 1973 Spängler et al.[11] described the use of fibrin sealant for full-thickness skin grafts in rats, and in 1977 Staindl[12,13] reported his clinical experiences using fibrin glue to seal skin grafts. The hemostatic effect and the high frequency of successful grafting have been pointed out as advantages. In 1979 Frey et al.[14] and in 1980 Rendl et al.[15] showed that fibrin-based sealing and grafting could even be achieved in infected wounds. Fibrin sealant was also used in punch hair grafting. Although it had no beneficial effect in routine punch hair transplantation, it was of some potential value if the grafts were left without any dressing immediately postoperatively.[16] In 1982 a fibrin sealant spray system was introduced[17] and successfully used for facelifts.[18]

According to Converse et al.,[19] a graft must be nourished by diffusion until vascularization starts on the third day. The netlike structure of physiologic fibrin sealants (forming a coarse, three-dimensional fibrin structure) allows diffusion into and nourishment of the graft during the first few days if it is applied in a thin layer. Furthermore, migration of cells and vascularization into the fibrin net starts on the third day after grafting. Histologic studies of fibrin-sealed split skin grafts were published by Braun et al.[20] in 1975 and by Spängler[21] in 1976. In burns, Fisseler-Eckhoff et al.[22] indicated that wound healing is accelerated for 12 days. Ten days after grafting, the fibrin sealant has been dissolved by fibrinolysis.

In 1988 Henrich et al.[23] compared the usefulness of three sealing systems in full-thickness skin grafts following burns. Their judgment was based on macroscopic criteria, and they concluded that two fibrin sealants were superior to cyanoacrylate.

A commercial fibrin sealant was first produced in 1978 from human plasma. It has proved to be effective in hemostasis, sealing of tissue, and wound healing. It is a two-component system. The first component, the sealer protein, contains highly concentrated fibrinogen and factor XIII in addition to other plasma proteins such as albumin and cold-insoluble globulin (fibronectin). The second component, the hardener, is a solution of thrombin and calcium chloride. A fibrinolysis inhibitor is generally added to one of the two components. This product may well be regarded as the conceptual prototype of fibrin sealant products now approved or under development.[24] More than 2000 papers have been published, and a good early overview on its action in the field was provided by two multivolume monographs in 1986 and 1994 by Schlag et al.[25,26] In memory of Schlag's pioneering role in the field, an award was established for the tissue sealant–trauma field in 1998.

When the two fibrin sealant components are mixed, coagulation occurs, and in the further course of the process, the activated factor XIII (factor XIIIa) causes cross-linking of the fibrin monomers.[27,28] After a few minutes, the fibrin γ-chains are completely cross-linked, whereas the process of fibrin α-chain cross-linking takes up to 2 hours with about 70% of maximum after 10 minutes. To achieve an optimum rate of cross-linking, $CaCl_2$ concentration must be ≥5 mmol/L.[29] An increasingly rigid clot is formed, which is gradually lysed and absorbed during the wound-healing process. The importance of fibrin cross-linking lies in the resulting increase in clot rigidity.[30] The elastic modulus, tensile strength, and adhesiveness are functions of fibrinogen concentration.[3,31] The importance of factor XIII in the fibrin sealant system, however, is not limited to fibrin cross-linking. The investigations of Duckert and Nyman[32] show that factor XIIIa also causes collagen to cross-link with fibrin, thus providing adhesive strength to tissues.

Factor XIIIa cross-links plasma-derived fibronectin to fibrin, which is important for cell adhesion via the RGD (Arg-Gly-Asp) domain.[33] Furthermore, α_2-antiplasmin and plasmin activator inhibitor 2 (PAI-2), which help to control subsequent fibrinolysis of the clot,[34] are also cross-linked to fibrin by factor XIIIa.

In a large-scale study comprising 11 cardiac surgery centers in the United States, Rousou et al.[35] were able to demonstrate that fibrin sealant could achieve hemostasis in a significantly shorter time than with any of the conventional methods. Other randomized studies also confirmed the excellent hemostatic effect of fibrin sealant in urology.[36] Kram et al.[37] corroborated the excellent hemostatic effect of fibrin sealant in spleen and liver surgical patients. On the basis of these clinical studies, Baxter-Immuno AG, Vienna, Austria, introduced commercial fibrin sealant as Tisseel to the U.S. market in 1998. The availability of commercial fibrin sealant varies geographically with Tisseel/Tissucol worldwide, Beriplast mainly in Europe and Japan, Hemaseel in the United States, Quixil mainly in the United Kingdom and Israel, and Bolheal in Japan. Several other fibrin sealants have been or are currently being developed.

Apart from highly concentrated fibrinogen from pooled plasma obtained via cryoprecipitation and further processing, fibrin-based sealants were also derived from single-donor or autologous sources.[38] Cryoprecipitate and autologous fibrin were found to have a low fibrinogen (clottable protein) concentration, only moderate α-chain cross-linking, and therefore only limited tensile strength.[39] With careful donor selection, screening (including polymerase chain reaction), and virus inactivation (heat or solvent/detergent, or both), commercial fibrin sealants have a longer than 20-year history of safety. Thus the demand for so-called home brews has decreased.[40] Such "homemade" sealants typically have less favorable sealing properties, similar to those of "platelet glue" sold in 1977 or a very high viscosity like HN-fraction, as a major drawback.[39,41,42]

Although, for example, commercial fibrin sealants were used together with bovine thrombin only until 1991 in Germany, bovine thrombin is still used with "home brews" or as free thrombin together with non-sealant–based hemostats like gelatin sponges. Large amounts of free bovine thrombin are considered a risk factor for formation of antibodies against bovine thrombin and factor V. These antibodies may cross-react with human thrombin and factor V, which in a worst case scenario can lead to disseminated intravascular coagulation.[43]

A variation of the standard fibrinogen-thrombin system has been introduced with the use of the snake venom enzyme batroxobin in 1997,[44] where acid-soluble fibrin I is formed first and then aggregated to a fibrin clot by increase of pH (alkaline buffer as the reaction partner in a two-component system).

For autologous (single-donor) fibrin sealant production, automatic processing apparatuses have been developed that are based on the batroxobin fibrin monomer approach (Vivostat, Vivolution A/S, Birkeroed, Denmark)[45] or on cryoprecipitation and further processing.[46] The latter (CryoSeal, ThermoGenesis Corp., Rancho Cordova, Calif.) has two separate channels for sealer protein and thrombin preparation, and was licensed as a device (CE Mark) in Europe in 1998. The CryoSeal uses an automated refrigeration device and also has the capability to make a human thrombin component.

In addition to plasma-derived products, fibrin sealant systems were also put together using recombinant components produced by transgenic sheep (fibrinogen in milk)[47] and cell cultures (prothrombin, factor XIII). The theoretical advantages, mainly the absence of human viruses, are overcome by the drawbacks including potential animal viruses and lack of other natural fibrin clot constituents (such as fibronectin and fibrin-bound growth factors) supporting wound healing.

In 1947 Ferry and Morrison[48] described the formation of two different kinds of fibrin clots: (1) white, nontransparent “coarse clots” formed at an ionic strength and pH value within the physiologic range, and (2) transparent “fine clots” produced at a higher ionic strength or pH value, or both. Fine clots are almost crystal clear and relatively brittle (Fig. 1-2). Transition from one type to the other is smooth, with fibrinogen concentration, thrombin concentration, and reaction temperature as further influencing factors. The tensile strength of coarse clots is significantly higher as shown by a 10-fold higher shear modulus.[49] The elastic rigidity measurements of fine clots revealed less than one tenth the shear modulus found for coarse clots. It is possible that the rigidity of the coarse clots is primarily due to steric immobilization, as has been suggested by Nelb et al.[50] The ionic strength of the fibrin sealant formulation can also affect the degree of cross-linking and cell toxicity (Fig. 1-2).[51,52]

Sealant degradation rate depends on:

1. The fibrinolytic (or more generally the proteolytic) activity in the area of application
2. The thickness of the sealant layer, which should be as thin as possible, since excessively long survival of the sealant may not be desirable[53]
3. The plasminogen content

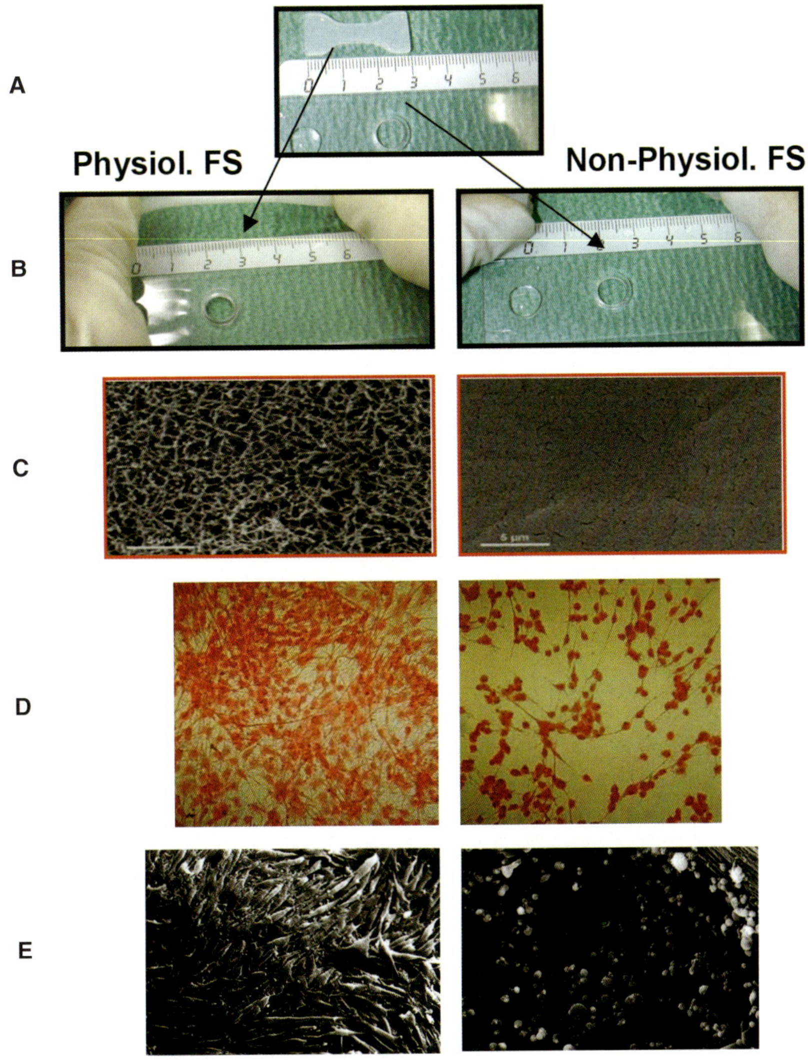

Figure 1-2 Comparison of coarse (physiologic) and fine (nonphysiologic) structures as obtained with different fibrin sealants. **A,** Macroscopic appearance: physiologic fibrin sealant turns opaque white upon coagulation, but nonphysiologic fibrin sealant remains clear. **B,** Elasticity: physiologic sealants have a high elasticity (length can increase up to twice the original), but nonphysiologic fine clots are brittle and break more easily when stretched. **C,** Ultrastructure: structure of fibrin sealant in the scanning electron microscope after fixation and critical point drying. Coarse structures similar to plasma clots are found in fibrin sealants with physiologic salt compositions, whereas a fine unphysiologic structure (almost no structure) is found in sealants with high salt content and other additives. **D,** Cytotoxicity: although physiologic sealant components have no effect on human fibroblasts in vitro, nonphysiologic sealants have a cytotoxic effect. **E,** Also, cells (MRC5 lung fibroblasts) do not spread and grow on the surface of nonphysiologic fine clots. (Experimental conditions are described in Redl et al.[52])

To a variable extent, sealant persistence in vivo can be controlled by adding an antifibrinolytic agent.[54] Studies have demonstrated that aprotinin, a natural protease inhibitor, is superior to synthetic antifibrinolytic agents.[55,56] Aprotinin has been added to many of the sealant systems to protect fibrin sealant from premature fibrinolytic/proteolytic degradation, because aprotinin was found to provide better stability than other protease inhibitors, for example, tranexamic acid (tAMCA).[29] Nevertheless, tAMCA has been included in one of the commercial fibrin sealant preparations, and in 2000 tAMCA incorporated into fibrin sealant was shown to cause convulsive seizures following subdural application in a rat model.[57] Therefore such sealants are contraindicated in the neurosurgical field. The causes of these convulsions were identified as a gamma-aminobutyric acid (GABA) receptor antagonistic effect.[58] Another approach to prevention of premature fibrinolysis was the removal of plasminogen from the fibrinogen component.[59] Because the proteolytic activity in wounds not only is related to plasminogen or plasminogen activator but also is largely dependent on leukocyte proteases, elastase or cathepsin G inhibitors could prevent premature clot lysis.[60]

Role of Fibrin in Wound Healing and Adhesion Prevention

Because mechanical union is just one aspect of successful surgery, wound-healing properties of sealants are also important. In 1960 Banerjee and Glynn[61] demonstrated that implanted fibrin clots are invaded by new capillaries and fibroblasts.

The formation of fibrin and its cross-linking by factor XIIIa are essential for wound healing. The fibrin network produced under physiologic conditions serves as a matrix for the ingrowth of fibroblasts and the formation of collagen fibers.[62,63] Dinges et al.[64] determined in a spongiosa-based granulation tissue model that fibrin sealant significantly stimulated fibroblast migration. Toriumi[65] determined in a pig tissue flap model that fibrin sealant provided more strength over the first 48 hours than was found in controls (no sealant).

In 1962 Beck et al.[66] found that factor XIII is essential for normal fibroblast proliferation. These findings were later confirmed and extended by other investigators.[67-69] According to Bruhn et al.,[70] fibroblast proliferation is stimulated by the presence of factor XIII, which at the same time has an inhibitory effect on epidermal cell proliferation.[71] According to Kasai et al.,[72] cross-linked fibrin rather than factor XIII as such is essential for cell proliferation.

The importance of fibrin in wound repair was confirmed by Brändstedt et al.[73] in studies on the impact of defibrination on wound healing. Fibrin is also essential for chemotaxis[74] of polymorphonuclear neutrophils (in vitro) because of its degradation products and its recruitment and activation of macrophages. Macrophages are an important part of the cell population in the wound because they contribute growth factors.

The effect of thrombin in wound healing is manifold and is a vital part of wound repair aside from its effects on platelet activation. Thrombin itself has mitogenic properties in cell cultures, such as a long-lasting hormone-like influence on fibroblast proliferation.[75] Furthermore, thrombin is involved in transformation of factor XIII to XIIIa, conversion of fibrinogen to fibrin, prostaglandin production, and activation of protein C.[76] Moreover, partial structures of thrombin act as nonproteolytically activated receptor (PPAR) agonist and improve wound healing.[77,78] The role of fibrin sealant in wound healing has been reviewed in more detail.[79]

In addition to wound healing, fibrin can have an impact on adhesion prevention. In 1984 Lindenberg and Lauritsen[80] reported for the first time that fibrin sealant can minimize postsurgical adhesions; this was partly challenged by others but was supported by further studies using modified fibrin sealant compositions.[81,82]

Preparation and Application of Fibrin Sealant

Although a high fibrinogen concentration is important for sealant strength, such a product, if lyophilized, is more difficult to dissolve in a lyophilized form. Therefore a special heating and stirring device was developed in 1980 (Fig. 1-3).[83] To partly overcome the slow dissolution without such a device, high-salt and other additions were included in some of the commercial fibrin sealant preparations, which, however, resulted in an unphysiologic fine clot structure (see Fig. 1-2). For user convenience a preassembled dual-syringe, deep-frozen system was also introduced in some of the markets, particularly in Europe in 1987.

Since the first applications of fibrin sealant, the strength obtainable has been known to depend both on the fibrinogen concentration[16] and on the amount of

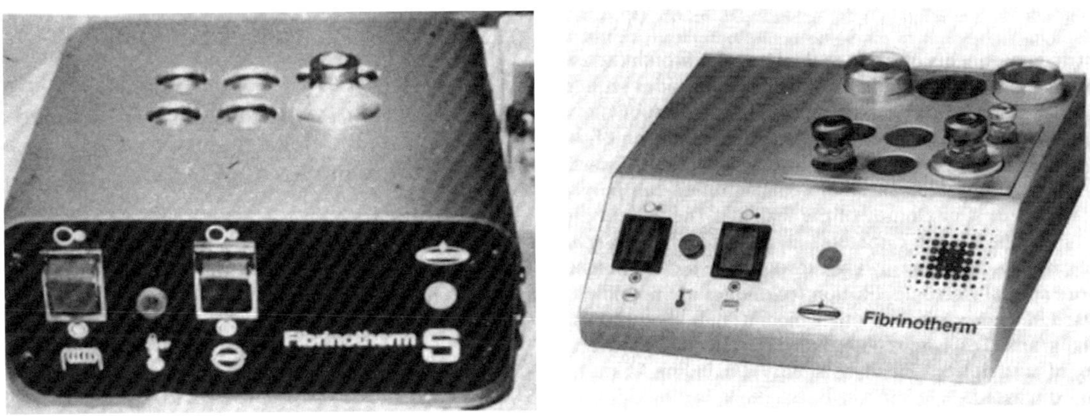

Figure 1-3 Two generations of a heater-stirrer device to speed up reconstitution of lyophilized fibrin sealant.

cross-linkage.[55] A design for measuring intrinsic clot strength[84] was used to determine an optimum mixing ratio. The mixture of one part sealant and one part thrombin solution produced the best results.[16]

Critics repeatedly have pointed out that the adhesive effect of fibrin sealant is not so strong as that of synthetics, for example, cyanoacrylate. This limited adhesive effect is, however, compensated for by its high elasticity,[39] which makes the fibrin sealant especially useful for nonstatic tissue, for example, skin grafts and lung parenchyma.

The classic application method involved the use of high thrombin concentrations (several 100 NIH U/ml) and consecutive application of the two components. This results in fast coagulation on the interface of the two components but subsequently also results in poor intermingling and poor rigidity of the resulting clot. Use of low thrombin concentrations (4 to 6 NIH U/ml) results in slow coagulation and allows premixing, which was introduced for nerve sealing.[85] A drawback of premixing is that it requires the surgeon to work quickly.

For these reasons an application device consisting of a double syringe and two detachable heads was developed in 1980.[16] The two components can be mixed and applied simultaneously, either through a needle or by spraying (Fig. 1-4). Both techniques are simple to use. High and low thrombin concentrations can be employed, and the two components are well mixed. Spraying in combination with a high thrombin concentration (500 NIH U/ml) has proved particularly effective in establishing hemostasis, whereas a low thrombin concentration (4 to 6 NIH U/ml) has proved beneficial in all applications where the parts to be sealed require subsequent adaptation, for example, in skin grafting and in some microsurgical operations for skin transplantation.[86] Especially in this application, a thin layer of fibrin sealant is the method of choice.[87]

In general, fibrin sealant can be sprayed with or without gas. Without gas the spray is usually more streaming or sprinkling than spraying if highly concentrated (and therefore more viscous) sealer protein solutions are used. The advantages are that the sprayer need not be tethered and no gas source is needed.

Spray systems with gas are connected to a conventional pressurized gas source (see Fig. 1-4).[16] Later on, similar application devices were introduced by other manufacturers. As the droplets bombard each other in the air and on the wound surface, they mix and at a high thrombin concentration instantly form a delicate fibrin film. A thin film produced in this manner is optimal to promote wound healing.[53] An additional advantage offered by spraying with gas is that the operating site can be cleaned and dried before application of the sealant. The sealant is thus applied to a "dry" surface, which improves its efficacy. Moreover, the device does not clog when the sealing procedure is interrupted. The spray head is especially useful for covering large areas, for example, for fixation of skin grafts and coating the donor area (Fig. 1-5).

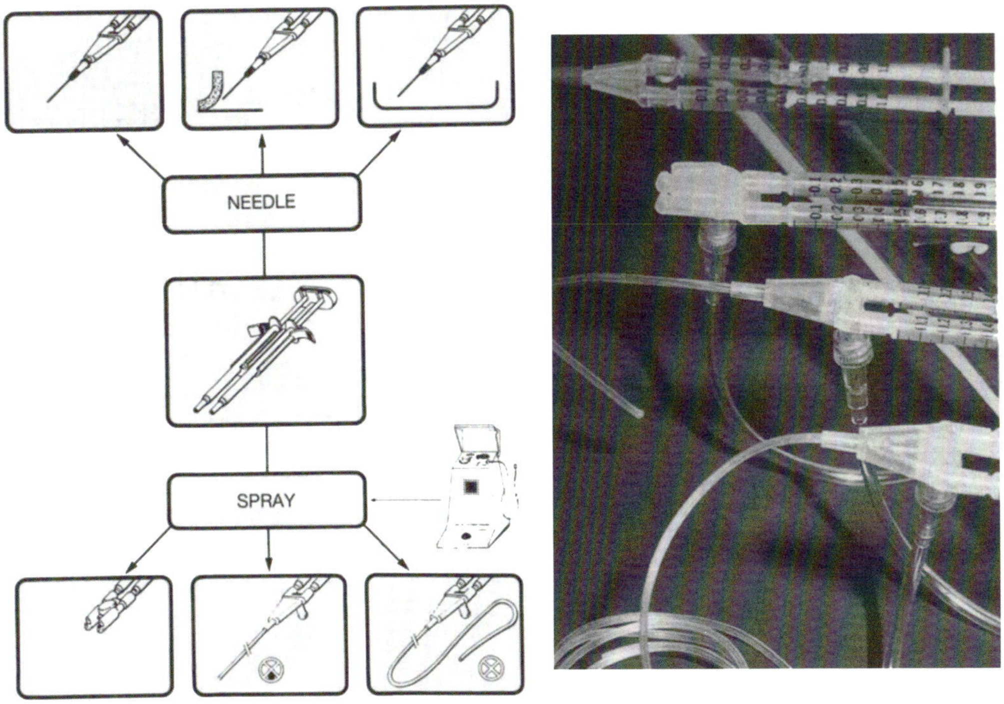

Figure 1-4 Several application devices or methods were described as early as 1980. (From Schlag G, Redl H, eds. Fibrin Sealant in Operative Medicine, vol. 3. Gynecology Obstetrics—Urology. Berlin: Springer-Verlag, 1986, pp 13-26.)

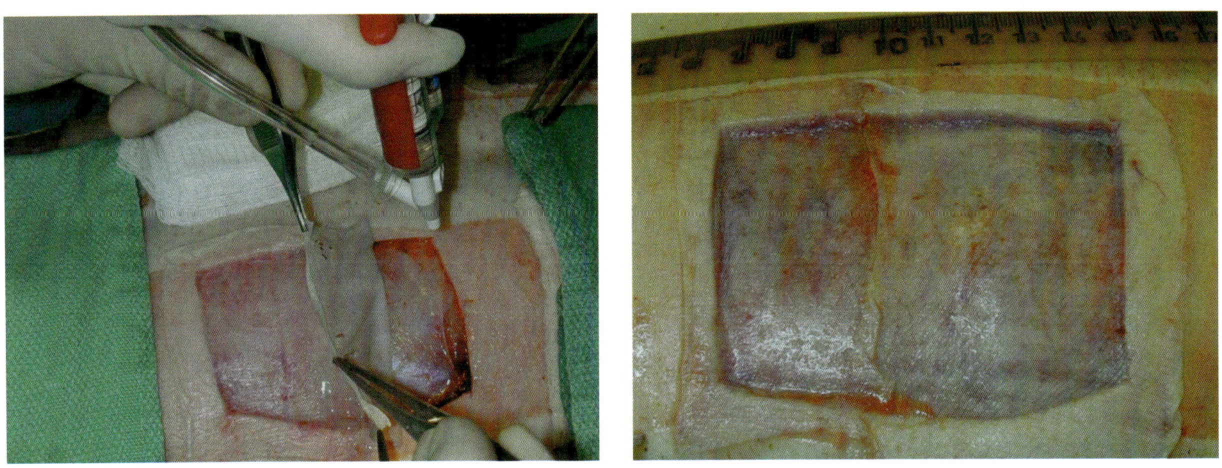

Figure 1-5 Optimal thin-layer spray application (with pressurized gas), introduced before 1980,[16] is especially well suited for skin transplantation (example from experimental study in pigs).

A four-lumen spray catheter (see Fig. 1-4) has also been introduced. Two lumens were used for the components, the third one for the gas, and in the short version a malleable wire is contained within the fourth lumen. Another version has been developed to seal otherwise inaccessible areas by endoscopy or with a malleable wire, which allows any specific catheter shape (see Fig. 1-4).[86] Unfortunately, it had to be withdrawn from the market because of adverse events caused by improper use. These catheters were used to successfully fix flaps in plastic surgery, for pleurodesis in recurrent pneumothorax,[88] to occlude bronchopleural,[89] rectovaginal, and esophageal bronchopleural fistulas,[90] to arrest gastric and esophageal bleeding, and to achieve hemostasis in epistaxis and after prostatectomy.

In addition to standard needle and spray application systems, specialized devices have been developed. Certain operations require the use of a microapplicator[86] that allows repeated application of the same small volume per ejection. This is especially useful with low thrombin concentrations (e.g., 4 NIH U/ml). A similar system was developed by Tange.[91] An alternative is to mix the two components on a piece of aluminum foil and apply the premixed sealant with a spatula.[92] The special device developed by Chüden[93] produced an "ultramicro" dosing (but without mixing). Furthermore, fibrin sealant has been used with a special biopsy and closure needle.[94]

Fibrin as a Biomatrix for Substances

The practice has been to apply fibrin sealant only to areas unlikely to become infected. To overcome this limitation, antibiotics were added to the fibrin sealant. As early as 1950, a patent was described in the United States in which the combination of fibrin and antibiotics was used.[95]

Antibiotics are released from fibrin seal by simple diffusion, which depends to a large extent on the concentration gradient between the clot and its environment. Although antibiotics incorporated into fibrin clots are retained longer than when they are directly instilled into body cavities, drug retention is much lower than with bone cement–antibiotic mixtures and is insufficient to maintain adequate local drug concentrations for more than a few days. Some antibiotics substantially inhibit the cross-linking reaction of fibrin. The rate of fibrin cross-linking in the presence of antibiotics can be normalized, however, by incorporating additional factor XIII (20 U/ml) into the reaction mixture.[55] Fibrin biomatrix has also been used in the delivery of chemotherapeutics such as 5-fluorouracil[96] or paclitaxel (Taxol).[97]

While fibrin-based biomatrix has been used as a cellular scaffold during wound healing, the efficacy can be enhanced by including bioactive agents that promote specific cellular responses. Certain growth factors, that is, basic fibroblast growth (bFGF) and vascular endothelial growth factor VEGF (only isoform 165) specifically bind to fibrin(ogen)[34,98] so that fibrin biomatrix can be directly used for delivery.[99] Delivering a combination of growth factors ($VEGF_{[165]}$ + $VEGF_{[121]}$) or ($VEGF_{[165]}$ + bFGF) constituted an improvement over the delivery of individual growth factors for enhancing neovascularization.[100]

Schwarz et al.[101] implanted allogenic demineralized bone powder and bone matrix gelatin with or without fibrin sealant in heterotopic and orthotopic sites in rats. Although fibrin sealant had no additional effect on bone induction, they noted that fibrin sealant facilitated application of smaller particles of bone-matrix gelatin and prevented hematoma formation. Further, it has been shown that a fibrin matrix supports handling and osteogenic properties of the ceramic materials including osteointegration, bone remodeling, and new bone formation.[102,103] Kawamura and Urist[104] used fibrin sealant to deliver partially purified bone morphogenetic protein and reported a synergistic effect. Although more intensive bone regeneration or more rapid fracture healing was achieved in a number of experiments by using fibrin sealant,[105-109] other investigators with different setups had negative results.[110-113] Zilch and Noffke[114] considered that delayed healing of such implants may have been caused by using too much fibrin sealant.

Fibrin as a Biomatrix for Cells

Use of keratinocytes combined with fibrin matrix was first described in 1988[115] for skin regeneration. When isolated keratinocytes are cultivated on a fibrin matrix, the relative percentage of epidermal stem cells found in vivo is maintained.[115] The autologous keratinocyte-fibrin approach also has been commercialized as Bioseed-S (Biotissue Technologies, Freiburg, Germany) in Europe. Furthermore, the use of fibrin microbeads is another approach to delivering cells, for example, fibroblasts for skin regeneration.[116]

Other cells including chondrocytes,[117] human myofibroblasts,[118] and osteoprogenitor cells[119] also have been successfully grown in fibrin gels. Moreover, fibrin sealant has been used to deliver tracheal epithelial cells and preadipocytes.[120]

The release of fibrinopeptide B from the β-chain of fibrinogen exposes a new N-terminal peptide domain on fibrin that serves as a unique binding site for the vascular endothelial (VE) cell surface receptor VE-cadherin.[121] Fibrin-specific signaling through this receptor causes the vascular endothelial cells in injured blood vessels to migrate, proliferate, differentiate, and form new blood capillaries. The fibrin clot then serves as the physical scaffold for this angiogenesis at the wound site. The resulting neovascularization is a prerequisite for successful tissue regeneration.[100]

Furthermore, a change in the concentration of the fibrinogen component and the thrombin component in the final fibrin clot produces a change in milieu. This change affects the cell behavior on and in these fibrin clots. For example, it has been shown that the way in which human monocytes, fibroblasts, keratinocytes, and mesenchymal and neuronal stem cells adhere and proliferate depends on the fibrin formulation.[122-126] In addition, the morphology of these cells is affected by the fibrin formulations. This change in cell behavior is also seen with human-derived fibroblasts incorporated within the three-dimensional physiologic network of coarse fibrin clots. For example, in fibrin formulations with high fibroblast proliferation, cells spread more than in fibrin formulations with low fibroblast proliferation.[127]

Combination of Fibrin With Collagen and Other Carriers

Fibrin sealants have frequently been used in combination with collagen fleeces.[56] Although not well suited for application in the cosmetic field, a fibrinogen-thrombin precoated collagen fleece (TachoComb, Nycomed Pharma AS, Asker, Norway) was introduced for hemostasis in 1990.[128] An absorbable bone sealant, Absele, has been used to control bleeding from the cut end of bone in neurosurgery. Absele was a paste made from stabilized fibrin and soluble collagen.[129] Fibrin was also used on a polylactide dressing (fibrin bandage) to achieve hemostasis.[130]

Collagen/Gelatin

In addition to the frequently used combinations of thrombin with cellulose and collagen-gelatin fleeces, collagen-based sealants (hemostats) have also been introduced. On the one hand, collagen fibers and thrombin were combined with autologous plasma (CoStasis, Cohesion Technologies, Inc., Palo Alto, Calif.).[131] On the other hand, partly cross-linked gelatin particles were combined with bovine thrombin to produce an effective hemostat that swells further on contact with blood and can even stop arterial bleeding (FloSeal, Baxter Corporation, Deerfield, Ill.). Its development, which began in 1996, culminated in successful clinical trials in 2000.[132] Both products are not widely used in cosmetic surgery.

Protein-Aldehyde Sealants

To overcome the limited tissue adhesiveness of fibrin sealant systems, several systems have been proposed that include covalent binding of proteins (bovine gelatin, bovine albumin) by means of aldehydes (formaldehyde, glutaraldehyde), which are well known for their tanning and tissue fixation properties in histology.

The gelatin-based resorcinol-formaldehyde glue was developed by Braunwald and Tatooles. A report on 12 years of experience with GRF for the treatment of aortic dissections was published in 1990.[133] GRF glue initially was reported to be free of significant associated risks, but later reports have suggested a danger of vascular tissue disruption.[134]

A bovine albumin–based glutaraldehyde cross-linked glue was developed and has been commercially available as BioGlue since 1998 (CE Mark) in Europe.

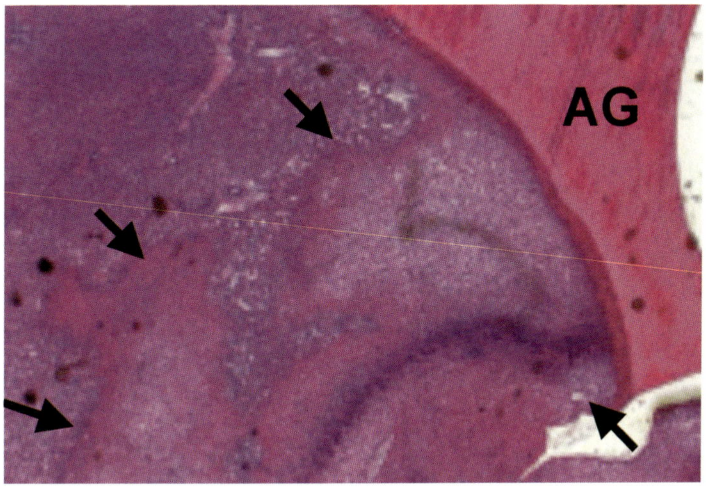

Figure 1-6 Severe necrosis *(arrows)* of the liver 48 hours after application of an albumin-glutaraldehyde sealant *(AG)* (experimental model in rabbits) (unpublished observations by H. Redl.)

Since 1999 the same product has been available in the United States under a Food and Drug Administration (FDA)–approved Humanitarian Device Exemption (HDE) for use as an adjunct to sutures and staples in the repair of acute thoracic dissections. Aside from its excellent bonding and easy storage and application characteristics, severe inflammatory responses have been reported[135] and corroborated in experimental studies (Fig. 1-6). This glue has a specific role in aortic dissection repairs and has been used successfully.[136] Albumin-glutaraldehyde glue can be used to eliminate the dissection plane by gluing the aortic layers together and strengthening the aortic support wall to suture more effectively.

Cyanoacrylate

Initial reports on these agents date back to 1949. They can be easily applied as a single-component glue system stored in a tube.[137] The adhesive properties of cyanoacrylate were described in 1959.[138] The cyanoacrylates were used clinically in 1965 by Watson and Maguda[139] for tympanic membrane repair. The glue is metabolized by hydrolysis to formaldehyde and alkylcyanoacetate, which can be further metabolized and excreted in urine and feces.[137] A cyanoacrylate (Histoacryl, B. Braun, Melsungen, Germany) was developed in an attempt to reduce tissue toxicity. The cytotoxicity of cyanoacrylate[140] is proportional to the dose used, and an association with liver sarcoma in animals has been reported.[141] N-butyl-cyanoacrylate agents have overcome some of these drawbacks and are especially well suited for skin closure. However, there have been case reports of complications following clinical use of cyanoacrylate agents.[142] Octyl-2-cyanoacrylate (Dermabond, Ethicon, Somerville, N.J.) has a slower rate of degradation and exhibits less inflammation. Octyl-2-cyanoacrylate is effective for superficial skin closure but should not be implanted subcutaneously.

Mussel Adhesive Protein

One of the exotic and also exciting materials is mussel adhesive protein, which allows the sea mussel *(Mytilus edulis)* to adhere to underwater surfaces.[143] It is a protein composed of repeats of hexapeptides and decapeptides containing high amounts of dihydroxyphenylalanine and 4-hydroxyproline[144] and has high adhesive strength because of these dopa residues. Although this adhesive is biodegradable and has been applied for chondrocyte fixation[145] and osteoblast fixation,[146] it is reported to have caused inflammatory responses upon intraocular injection[147] and is presently limited to laboratory use only.

Polyethylene Glycol–Based/Associated Sealants

No literature accessible by Medline has been published on the use of PEG-related tissue sealants in cosmetic or reconstructive surgery. Its main usage areas are lung parenchyma and graft anastomosis sealing. No direct support of wound regeneration as achieved with fibrin-based material is to be expected.

In principal, two reactive PEG components polymerize in situ upon mixing in the applicator tip and at the tissue surface to form an elastic hydrogel, commercially available as CoSeal (Cohesion Technologies, Inc., Palo Alto, Calif.). The reactive PEGs are quadrupolic PEG molecules with four reactive groups, either N-hydroxy succinimide or thiol. Under moderate alkaline pH conditions, these reactive groups form thioester cross-links with each other and covalent bonds with tissue amino groups. These covalent bonds achieve good tissue adhesion. The sealant is formed by simultaneously spraying two dissolved polymers directly onto, for example, suture lines. The combined polymers rapidly gel (within 5 seconds) and set within 60 seconds. This system has been successfully used for treatment of suture line bleeding in an iliac polytetrafluoroethylene graft model[148] and received FDA (device route) approval in 2002.

In 2000 the FDA approved a type of light-activated PEG-based surgical sealant for use in lungs to seal air leaks following removal of cancerous lung tumors. The sealant FocalSeal-L (Genzyme Biosurgery, Cambridge, Mass.) is applied to tissue, which has to be pretreated with a conditioner. Activated by light, the product forms a sealant via chemical and photochemical polymerization processes. Studies in 180 patients showed that 39% of patients treated with FocalSeal-L and standard techniques remained free of air leaks until they were discharged from the hospital compared to 11% of patients treated with standard techniques alone. There was a higher incidence of infection in patients treated with FocalSeal-L (7.2% vs. 3.6%).[149]

The combination of albumin and succinylated PEG has been used as a sealant especially for lung parenchyma and suture lines.[150]

Conclusion

Many different tissue sealants or hemostats have been developed over the past 30 years since the successful reintroduction of fibrin by Helene Matras. Each one has certain advantages and specific areas of application. Three such different systems (classic fibrin sealant, gelatin particle–thrombin, and PEG-based materials) are currently available from one vendor, for example.

Tissue sealants not only have a long history, but a bright future as well. Fibrin sealants are additionally used as a biomatrix and scaffold, for example, for stem cells and growth factors or plasmids. The bright future of tissue sealants might also include new technologies such as self-assembling nanostructures.

ACKNOWLEDGMENTS

This review is dedicated to our former collaborators, who contributed enormously to this field: Helene Matras, Heinz Kuderna, Hans Dinges, Günther Schlag, and Thomas Seelich. We also want to acknowledge William D. Spotnitz's excellent work regarding the history of tissue sealants, which has been a valuable resource for this review.

We thank Bill Tawil, Thomas Seelich, and Walter Fuerst for critical reading and supplementing as well as Linda Pelinka for language revision. This review is also dedicated to our fantastic sealant investigation team lead by Manuela Simunek and Walter Fuerst.

REFERENCES

1. Majno G. Healing Hand—Man and Wound in the Ancient World. Cambridge, Mass: Harvard University Press, 1999.
2. Spotnitz WD. History of tissue adhesives. In Sierra D, Saltz R, eds. Surgical Adhesives and Sealants. Current Technology and Applications. Basel: Technomic Publishing, 1996.
3. Sierra DH. Fibrin sealant adhesive systems: A review of their chemistry, material properties and clinical applications. J Biomater Appl 7:309-352, 1993.
4. Bergel S. Über die Wirkung des Fibrins [About the effects of fibrin]. Dtsch Med Wochenschr 663-665, 1909.
5. Tidrick RT, Warner J. Fibrin fixation of skin transplants. Surgery 15:90-95, 1944.
6. Cronkite EP, Lozner EL, Deaver JM. Use of thrombin and fibrinogen in skin grafting. JAMA 124:976-978, 1944.
7. Bering EA Jr. Chemical, clinical and immunological studies on the products of human plasma fractionation. XX. The development of fibrin foam as hemostatic agent and for use in conjunction with human thrombin. J Clin Invest 23:586-590, 1944.
8. Gerendás M. Fibrin products as aids in hemostasis and wound healing. In Laki K, ed. Fibrinogen. New York: Marcel Dekker, 1968.
9. Matras H, Dinges HP, Lassmann H, Mamoli B. Zur nahtlosen interfaszikulären Nerventransplantation im Tierexperiment. [Suture-free interfascicular nerve transplantation in animal experiments]. Wien Med Wochenschr 122:517-523, 1972.
10. Kuderna H. Klinische Anwendung der Klebung von Nervenanastomosen mit Fibrinogen. [Clinical application of nerve-anastomoses sealing using fibrinogen]. Fortschr Kiefer Gesichtschir 21:135, 1976.
11. Spängler HP Jr, Holle J, Braun F. Gewebeklebung mit Fibrin. [Tissue sealing with fibrin]. Wien Klin Wochenschr 85:827-829, 1973.

12. Staindl O. Die Gewebeklebung mit hochkonzentriertem, humanem Fibrinogen am Beispiel der freien autologen Hauttransplantation. [Tissue sealing using highly concentrated human fibrinogen on the example of free, autologous skin-grafting]. Arch Otorhinolaryngol 217:219-228, 1977.
13. Staindl O. Indications of the fibrin sealant in facial plastic surgery. Facial Plast Surg 2:323-340, 1985.
14. Frey M, Holle J, Mandl H, Freilinger G. Die Vorteile der aufgeschobenen Spalthautlappentransplantation und die Erweiterung ihres Anwendungsbereiches durch die Verwendung des Fibrinklebers. [Advantages of delayed split skin transplantation and widened usage due to use of fibrin sealant]. Acta Chir Austriaca 5:97-100, 1979.
15. Rendl KH, Staindl O, Zelger J, Chmelicek-Feurstein C. Die Hauttransplantation mit Fibrinkleber beim Ulcus cruris. [Skin transplantation with fibrin sealant]. Aktuelle Dermatol 6:199-203, 1980.
16. Nordstrom RE, Piechotta UF, Flemming I. Fibrin sealant in punch hair grafting. J Dermatol Surg Oncol 13:1009-1011, 1987.
17. Redl H, Schlag G, Dinges HP. Methods of fibrin seal application. Thorac Cardiovasc Surg 30:223-227, 1982.
18. Marchac D, Sandor G. Face lifts and sprayed fibrin glue: An outcome analysis of 200 patients. Br J Plast Surg 47:306-309, 1994.
19. Converse JM, Uhlschmidt GK, Ballantyne DL. Plasmacirculation. Plast Reconstr Surg 43:495, 1969.
20. Braun VF, Holle J, Kovac W, Lindner A, Spängler HP. Untersuchungen über die Replantation autologer Vollhaut mit Hilfe von hochkonzentriertem Fibrinogen und Blutgerinnungsfaktor XIII. [Studies on the replantation of autologous full-thickness skin grafts using highly concentrated fibrinogen and clotting factor XIII]. Wien Med Wochenschr 125:213-219, 1975.
21. Spängler HP. Gewebeklebung und lokale Blutstillung mit Fibrinogen, Thrombin und Blutgerinnungsfaktor XIII (experimentelle Untersuchungen und klinische Erfahrungen). [Tissue adhesion and local haemostasis using fibrinogen, thrombin and clotting factor XIII. (experimental investigations—clinical experience)]. Wien Klin Wochenschr Suppl 49: 3-18, 1976.
22. Fisseler-Eckhoff A, Grabosch A, Donati I, Müller KM. Histologische Untersuchungsergebnisse nach Hauttransplantation mit und ohne Fibrinkleber. [Histological results after skin transplantation with and without fibrin sealant]. Ellipse 15:180-186, 1988.
23. Henrich HA, Bäumer F, Oberschelp J, Kilian K. Einfluss von drei verschiedenen Gewebeklebern auf Vollhauttransplantate bei Verbrennungen. [Influence of three different tissue sealants of full-thickness skin transplants in burns]. Med Welt 39:701-706, 1981.
24. Jackson MR, MacPhee MJ, Drohan WN, Alving BM. Fibrin sealant: Current and potential clinical applications. Blood Coagul Fibrinolysis 7:737-746, 1996.
25. Schlag G, Redl H. Fibrin Sealant in Operative Medicine. Berlin: Springer-Verlag, 1986.
26. Schlag G, Redl H. Fibrin Sealing in Surgical and Nonsurgical Fields. Berlin: Springer-Verlag, 1994.
27. Laki K. Fibrinoligase: The fibrin-stabilizing factor system of blood plasma. Ann N Y Acad Sci 202:6-30, 1972.
28. Schwartz ML, Pizzo SV, Hill RL, McKee PA. Human factor XIII from plasma and platelets. Molecular weights, subunit structures, proteolytic activation, and cross-linking of fibrinogen and fibrin. J Biol Chem 248:1395-1407, 1973.
29. Seelich T, Redl H. Das Fibrinklebesystem. Biochemische Grundlagen der Klebemethode. [The fibrin sealant system. Biochemical background of the sealing method]. Dtsch Z Mund-Kiefer-Gesichts-Chir 3:22-26, 1979.
30. Shen LL, McDonagh RP, McDonagh J, Hermans J Jr. Fibrin gel structure. Influence of calcium and covalent cross-linking on the elasticity. Biochem Biophys Res Commun 56:793-798, 1974.

31. Khare A, Woo L, McLean A, Helgerson S. Mechanical characterization of fibrin gels. Blood Coagul Fibrinolysis 9:105, 1998.
32. Duckert F, Nyman D. Factor XIII, fibrin and collagen. In Gastpar H, ed. Collagen-Platelet Interaction, Proceedings of the First Munich Symposium on Biology of Connective Tissue, July 1976. Stuttgart–New York: F. K. Schattauer, 1978.
33. Danen EH, Yamada KM. Fibronectin, integrins, and growth control. J Cell Physiol 189:1-13, 2001.
34. Mosesson MW, Siebenlist KR, Meh DA. The structure and biological features of fibrinogen and fibrin. Ann N Y Acad Sci 936:11-30, 2001.
35. Rousou J, Levitsky S, Gonzalez-Lavin L, Cosgrove D, Magilligan D, Weldon C, Hiebert C, Hess P, Joyce L, Bergsland J. Randomized clinical trial of fibrin sealant in patients undergoing resternotomy or reoperation after cardiac operations. A multicenter study. J Thorac Cardiovasc Surg 97:194-203, 1989.
36. Gasser G, Mossig H, Fischer M, Eidler R, Klaring W, Lurf H. Modifikation der suprapubischen Prostatektomie unter Verwendung eines biologsichen Klebeverfahrens. [Modification of suprapubic prostatectomy using a biological gluing technic]. Wien Klin Wochenschr 95:399-403, 1983.
37. Kram HB, Reuben BI, Fleming AW, Shoemaker WC. Use of fibrin glue in hepatic trauma. J Trauma 28:1195-1201, 1988.
38. Saltz R, Sierra D, Feldman D, Saltz MB, Dimick A, Vasconez LO. Experimental and clinical applications of fibrin glue. Plast Reconstr Surg 88:1005-1015, 1991.
39. Redl H, Schlag G. Properties of different tissue sealants with special emphasis on fibrinogen based preparations. In Schlag G, Redl H, eds. Fibrin Sealant in Operative Medicine, vol. 3: Gynaecology and Obstetrics—Urology. Berlin: Springer-Verlag, 1986.
40. Mintz PD, Mayers L, Avery N, Flanagan HL, Burks SG, Spotnitz WD. Fibrin sealant: clinical use and the development of the University of Virginia Tissue Adhesive Center. Ann Clin Lab Sci 31:108-118, 2001.
41. Hamm KD, Beer R. Klebefestigkeitsuntersuchungen an biologischen Gewebeklebern. [Studies on the adhesive strength of biological tissue sealants]. Z Exp Chir Transplant Künstliche Organe 18:281-288, 1985.
42. Silverberg GD, Harbury CB, Rubenstein E. A physiological sealant for cerebrospinal fluid leaks. J Neurosurg 46:215-219, 1977.
43. Schoenecker JG, Hauck RK, Mercer MC, Parker W, Lawson JH. Exposure to topical bovine thrombin during surgery elicits a response against the xenogeneic carbohydrate galactose alpha1-3galactose. J Clin Immunol 20:434-444, 2000.
44. Dascombe WH, Dumanian G, Hong C, Heil BV, Labadie K, Hessel B, Blombaeck B, Johnson PC. Application of thrombin based fibrin glue and non-thrombin based batroxobin glue on intact human blood vessels: Evidence for transmural thrombin activity. Thromb Haemost 78:947-951, 1997.
45. Kjaergard HK, Trumbull HR. Vivostat system autologous fibrin sealant: Preliminary study in elective coronary bypass grafting. Ann Thorac Surg 66:482-486, 1998.
46. Gosselin RC, Larkin E, Owings JT, Coehlo P. CryoSeal system, a new device for generating cryoprecipitate from plasma. Clin Chem 43:1782-1783, 1997.
47. Butler SP, van Cott K, Subrumanian A, Gwazduaskas FC, Velander WH. Current progress in the production of recombinant human fibrinogen in the milk of transgenic animals. Thromb Haemost 78:537-542, 1997.
48. Ferry JD, Morrison PR. Preparation and properties of serum and plasma proteins.VIII. The conversion of human fibrinogen to fibrin under various conditions. J Am Chem Soc 69:388-400, 1947.
49. Kamykowski GW, Mosher DF, Lorand L, Ferry JD. Modification of shear modulus and creep compliance of fibrin clots by fibronectin. Biophys Chem 13:25-28, 1981.
50. Nelb GW, Gerth C, Ferry JD. Rheology of fibrin clots. III. Shear creep and creep recovery of fine ligated and coarse unligated clots. Biophys Chem 5:377-387, 1976.

51. Seelich T. Tissucol (Immuno, Vienna): Biochemistry and methods of application. J Head Neck Pathol 3:65-69, 1982.
52. Redl H, Schlag G, Dinges HP. Vergleich zweier Fibrinkleber. Einfluss ionischer Zusätze auf Fibrinstruktur sowie Morphologie und Wachstum menschlicher Fibroblasten. [Comparison of two fibrin sealants. Influence of ionic additives on fibrin structure as well as morphology and growth of human fibroblasts]. Med Welt 36:769-776, 1985.
53. Schlag G, Redl H, Thurnher M, Dinges HP. The importance of fibrin in wound repair. In Schlag G, Redl H, eds. Principles of Fibrin Sealant. Berlin: Springer-Verlag, 1986.
54. Pflueger H, Redl H. Abbau von Fibrin-Kleber in vivo und in vitro (Versuche an der Ratte). [In vivo and in vitro degradation of fibrin adhesives (studies in rats)]. Z Urol Nephrol 75:25-30, 1982.
55. Redl H, Schlag G, Dinges HP, Kuderna H, Seelich T. Background and methods of fibrin sealing. In Winter GD, Gibbons DF, Plenk H Jr, eds. Biomaterials 1980. New York: John Wiley & Sons, 1982.
56. Stemberger A, Fritsche HM, Haas S, Spilker G, Wriedt-Lübbbe I, Blümel G. Biochemische und experimentelle Aspekte der Gewebeversiegelung mit Fibrinogen und Kollagen. [Biochemical and experimental aspects of tissue sealing with fibrinogen and collagen]. In Cotta H, Braun A, eds. Fibrinkleber in Orthopädie und Traumatologie. Stuttgart, New York: Georg Thieme Verlag, 1982.
57. Schlag MG, Hopf R, Redl H. Convulsive seizures following subdural application of fibrin sealant containing tranexamic acid in a rat model. Neurosurgery 47:1463-1467, 2000.
58. Furtmuller R, Schlag MG, Berger M, Hopf R, Huck S, Sieghart W, Redl H. Tranexamic acid, a widely used antifibrinolytic agent, causes convulsions by a gamma-aminobutyric acid (A) receptor antagonistic effect. J Pharmacol Exp Ther 301:168-173, 2002.
59. Tse DC, Liu SL, Alpern M, Mankarious SS, Thomas WR, Enomoto S, and Garanchon CM. Topical fibrinogen complex. Patent USSN 08/632.922, 1997.
60. Redl H, Schlag G, Eibl J. Gewebekleber. Patent AT406120B, 1997.
61. Banerjee SK, Glynn LE. Reactions to homologous and heterologous fibrin implants in experimental animals. Ann N Y Acad Sci 1054-1057, 1960.
62. Ross R. The fibroblast and wound repair. Biol Rev 43:51-96, 1968.
63. Beck E, Duckert F, Vogel A, Ernst M. The influence of fibrin stabilizing factor on the growth of fibroblasts in vitro and wound healing. Thromb Diath Haemorrh 6:485-491, 1961.
64. Dinges HP, Redl H, Thurnher M, Schiesser A, Schlag G. Morphometric studies on wound healing after systemic administration of adriamycin and local application of fibrin sealant. Application of a new wound healing model using spongiosa implants. Pathol Res Pract 181:746-754, 1986.
65. Toriumi D. Surgical tissue adhesives: Host tissue response, adhesive strength and clinical performance. In Sierra D, Saltz R, eds. Surgical Adhesives and Sealants. Current Technology and Applications. Basel: Technomic Publishing, 1996.
66. Beck E, Duckert F, Vogel A, Ernst M. Der Einfluss des fibrinstabilisierenden Faktors (FSF) auf Funktion und Morphologie von Fibroblasten in vitro. [The influence of a fibrin stabilizing factor on function and morphology of fibroblasts in vitro]. Z Zellforschung 57:327-346, 1962.
67. Bruhn HD, Christophers E, Pohl J, Scholl G. Regulation der Fibroblastenproliferierung durch Fibrinogen, Fibrin, Fibronectin und Faktor XIII. [Regulation of fibroblast proliferation by fibrinogen, fibrin, fibronectin and factor XIII]. In Schimpf K, ed. Fibrinogen, Fibrin und Fibrinkleber. Stuttgart: Schattauer-Verlag, 1980.
68. Turowski G, Schaadt M, Barthels M, Diehl V, Poliwada H. Unterschiedlicher Einfluss von Fibrinogen und Faktor XIII auf das Wachstum von Primär- und Kulturfibroblasten. [Different influence of fibrinogen and factor XIII on the growth of primary and cultivated fibroblasts]. In Schimpf K, ed. Fibrinogen, Fibrin und Fibrinkleber. Stuttgart: Schattauer-Verlag, 1980.

69. Knoche H, Schmitt G. Autoradiographische Untersuchungen über den Einfluss des Faktors XIII auf die Wundheilung im Tierexperiment. [Autoradiographic investigation into the influence of factor XIII on wound healing in the animal experiment]. Arzneimittelforschung 26:547-551, 1976.
70. Bruhn HD, Pohl J. Growth regulation of fibroblasts by thrombin, factor XIII and fibronectin. Klin Wochenschr 59:145-146, 1981.
71. Hashimoto T, Marks R. Factor XIII inhibits epidermal cell migration in vitro. J Invest Dermatol 83:441-444, 1984.
72. Kasai S, Kunimoto T, Nitta J. Cross-link of fibrin by activated factor XIII stimulated attachment, morphological changes and proliferation of fibroblasts. Biomed Res 4: 155-160, 1983.
73. Brändstedt S, Rank F, Olson PS. Wound healing and formation of granulation tissue in normal and defibrinogenated rabbits. An experimental model and histological study. Eur Surg Res 12:12-21, 1980.
74. Key AB, Pepper DS, Ewart MR. Generation of chemotactic activity for leukocytes by the action of thrombin on human fibrinogen. Nature 243:56-57, 1973.
75. Pohl J, Bruhn HD, Christophers E. Thrombin and fibrin-induced growth of fibroblasts: Role in wound repair and thrombus organization. Klin Wochenschr 57:273-277, 1979.
76. Gustafson GT. Ecology of wound healing in the oral cavity. Scand J Haematol Suppl 40:393-409, 1984.
77. Carney DH, Mann R, Redin WR, Pernia SD, Berry D, Heggers JP, Hayward PG, Robson MC, Christie J, Annable C. Enhancement of incisional wound healing and neovascularization in normal rats by thrombin and synthetic thrombin receptor-activating peptides. J Clin Invest 89:1469-1477, 1992.
78. Stiernberg J, Redin WR, Warner WS, Carney DH. The role of thrombin and thrombin receptor activating peptide (TRAP-508) in initiation of tissue repair. Thromb Haemost 70:158-162, 1993.
79. Amrani DL, DiOrio JP, Delmotte Y. Wound healing. Role of commercial fibrin sealants. Ann N Y Acad Sci 936:566-579, 2001.
80. Lindenberg S, Lauritsen JG. Prevention of peritoneal adhesion formation by fibrin sealant. An experimental study in rats. Ann Chir Gynaecol 73:11-13, 1984.
81. Delmotte Y, Krack G. Self-supporting sheet-like material of cross-linked fibrin for preventing postoperative adhesion. Patent WO 96/22115, 1996.
82. Redl H. Fibrinogen plus a non-plasmin-acting fibrinolysis inhibitor for the reduction or prevention of adhesion formation. Patent WO 02/30445 A2, 2002.
83. Redl H, Seelich T. Verfahren und Vorrichtung zur Beschleunigung des Auflösens von schwerlöslichen lyophilisierten Arzneimitteln. [Method and apparatus for the accelerated solubilization of a difficult to dissolve lyophilized medication]. Patent AT4289/80, 1980.
84. Redl H, Stanek G, Hirschl A, Schlag G. Fibrinkleber-Antibiotika-Gemische-Festigkeit und Elutionsverhalten. [Fibrin sealant–antibiotics mixtures—strength and elution characteristics]. In Cotta H, Braun A, eds. Fibrinkleber in Orthopädie und Traumatologie. Stuttgart, New York: Georg Thieme Verlag, 1982.
85. Kuderna H. Das Fibrinklebesystem-Nervenklebung. [The fibrin sealant system—sealing of nerves]. Dtsch Z Mund-Kiefer-Gesichts-Chir 3:32-35, 1979.
86. Redl H, Schlag G. Fibrin sealant and its modes of application. In Schlag G, Redl H, eds. Fibrin Sealant in Operative Medicine, vol. 3: Gynaecology and Obstetrics—Urology. Berlin: Springer-Verlag, 1986.
87. O'Grady KM, Agrawal A, Bhattacharyya TK, Shah A, Toriumi DM. An evaluation of fibrin tissue adhesive concentration and application thickness on skin graft survival. Laryngoscope 110:1931-1935, 2000.
88. Jessen C, Sharma P. Use of fibrin glue in thoracic surgery. Ann Thorac Surg 39:521-524, 1985.

89. Waclawiczek HW, Chmelizek F. Endoscopic occlusion of bronchus stump fistulae following pneumonectomy with fibrin sealant in animal experiments. In Schlag G, Redl H, eds. Fibrin Sealant in Operative Medicine, vol. 5: Thoracic Surgery—Cardiovascular Surgery. Berlin: Springer-Verlag, 1986.
90. Flicker M, Pesendorfer FX, Redl H. Verschluss einer bronchoösophagealen Fistel. [Closure of a bronchopleural fistula]. Wr Med Wochenschr 135(Suppl 90):21-22, 1985.
91. Tange RA. A new application method for fibrin sealant: The glue gun. In Schlag G, Redl H, eds. Fibrin Sealant in Operative Medicine, vol. 1: Otorhinolaryngology, Berlin: Springer-Verlag, 1986.
92. Redl H, Schlag G. Background and methods of fibrin sealing. In Skjoldborg H, ed. Scientific Workshop '82: Tisseel/Tissucol Symposium—Areas of Application, Problems and Perspectives in Current Surgery. Immuno Denmark, 1984.
93. Chüden HG. Simplified application of fibrinous glue in middle-ear surgery. In Schlag G, Redl H, eds. Fibrin Sealant in Operative Medicine, vol. 1: Otorhinolaryngology. Berlin: Springer-Verlag, 2003.
94. Zatloukal K, Dinges HP, Thurnher M, Redl H, Schlag G. A new technique of liver biopsy with plugging of the needle track using a double channel biopsy device. An experimental study. Z Gastroenterol 26:699-703, 1988.
95. Ferry JD, Morrison PR. Fibrin clots and methods for preparing the same. Patent 2,533,004, 5-12-1950.
96. Yoshida H, Yamaoka Y, Shinoyama M, Kamiya A. Novel drug delivery system using autologous fibrin glue–release properties of anti-cancer drugs. Biol Pharm Bull 23:371-374, 2000.
97. MacPhee MJ, Singh MP, Brady R Jr, Akhyani N, Liau G, Lasa C Jr, Hue C, Best A, Drohan W. Fibrin sealant: A versatile delivery vehicle for drugs and biologics. In Sierra D, Saltz R, eds. Surgical Adhesives and Sealants. Current Technology and Applications. Basel: Technomic Publishing, 1996.
98. Sahni A, Francis CW. Vascular endothelial growth factor binds to fibrinogen and fibrin and stimulates endothelial cell proliferation. Blood 96:3772-3778, 2000.
99. Hasimoto J, Kurosaka M, Yoshiya S, Hirohata K. Meniscal repair using fibrin sealant and endothelial cell growth factor. Am J Sports Med 20:537-541, 1992.
100. Wong C, Inman E, Spaethe R, Helgerson S. Fibrin-based biomaterials to deliver human growth factors. Thromb Haemost 89:573-582, 2003.
101. Schwarz N, Redl H, Schlag G, Schiesser A, Lintner F, Dinges HP, Thurnher M. The influence of fibrin sealant on demineralized bone matrix–dependent osteoinduction. A quantitative and qualitative study in rats. Clin Orthop 238:282-287, 1989.
102. Daculsi G, Bagot d'Arc M, Cottreal M. Calcium phosphate ceramics (triosite) in otology: Evaluation in animals and application in humans. In Schlag G, Redl H, eds. Fibrin Sealing in Surgical and Nonsurgical Fields, vol. 1: Wound Healing. Berlin: Springer-Verlag, 1994.
103. Bagot d'Arc M, Corlieu P, Daculsi G. Mastoid cavity filling for bone reconstruction with a mixture of fibrin glue and ceramic granules. In Schlag G, Redl H, eds. Fibrin Sealant in Surgical and Nonsurgical Fields, vol. 5: Neurosurgery, Ophthalmic Surgery, ENT. Berlin: Springer-Verlag, 1994.
104. Kawamura M, Urist MR. Human fibrin is a physiologic delivery system for bone morphogenetic protein. Clin Orthop 235:302-310, 1988.
105. Boehler N, Boesch P, Sandbach G, Schlag G, Eschberger J, Schmid L. Der Einfluss von homologem Fibrinogen auf die Osteotomieheilung beim Kaninchen. [The influence of homologous fibrinogen on osteotomy healing in rabbits]. Unfallheilkunde 80:501-508, 1977.
106. Boesch P, Braun F, Eschberger J, Kovac W, Spaengler HP. Die Beeinflussung der Knochenheilung durch hochkonzentriertes Fibrin. Untersuchungen am Kaninchen. [The action of high concentrations of fibrin on bone healing]. Arch Orthop Unfallchir 89:259-273, 1977.

107. Boesch P, Lintner F, Arbes H, Brand G. Experimental investigations of the effect of the fibrin adhesive on the Kiel heterologous bone graft. Arch Orthop Trauma Surg 96:177-185, 1980.
108. Palacios-Carvajal J, Moina EM. The mixture of fibrin sealant and a porous ceramic as osteoconductor. In Schlag G, Redl H, eds. Fibrin Sealant in Operative Medicine, vol. 7: Traumatology—Orthopaedics. Berlin: Springer-Verlag, 1986.
109. Wischhoefer E, Hellerer O, Falter E, Hertlein H. Verhalten autologer Beckenkammspongiosa nach Transplantation mit und ohne Fibrinklebesystem in der Femurepiphyse des Hundes. [The behaviour of autologous spongiosa transplants from the ilial crest with and without fibrin adhesive in the canine femoral epiphysis]. Unfallheilkunde 85:250-252, 1982.
110. Albrektsson T, Bach A, Edshage S, Jonsson A. Fibrin adhesive system (FAS) influence on bone healing rate: A microradiographical evaluation using the bone growth chamber. Acta Orthop Scand 53:757-763, 1982.
111. Greco F, de Palma L, Specchia N, Lisai P. Experimental investigation into reparative osteogenesis with fibrin adhesive. Arch Orthop Trauma Surg 107:99-104, 1988.
112. Lucht U, Bunger C, Moller JT, Joyce F, Plenk H Jr. Fibrin sealant in bone transplantation. No effects on blood flow and bone formation in dogs. Acta Orthop Scand 57:19-24, 1986.
113. Zilch H. Der Einfluss des Fibrinklebers auf die Revaskularisierung des Knochentransplantates. [The influence of the fibrinogen adhesive system on revascularization of bone graft]. Unfallheilkunde 84:353-362, 1981.
114. Zilch H, Noffke B. Der Einfluss des Fibrinklebers auf die Knochenheilung. [The influence of the fibrinogen adhesive system on bone healing]. Unfallheilkunde 84:363-372, 1981.
115. Hunyadi J, Farkas B, Bertenyi C, Olah J, Dobozy A. Keratinocyte grafting: A new means of transplantation for full-thickness wounds. J Dermatol Surg Oncol 14:75-78, 1988.
116. Gorodetsky R, Clark RA, An J, Gailit J, Levdansky L, Vexler A, Berman E, Marx G. Fibrin microbeads (FMB) as biodegradable carriers for culturing cells and for accelerating wound healing. J Invest Dermatol 112:866-872, 1999.
117. van Susante JL, Buma P, Schuman L, Homminga GN, van den Berg WB, Veth RP. Resurfacing potential of heterologous chondrocytes suspended in fibrin glue in large full-thickness defects of femoral articular cartilage: An experimental study in the goat. Biomaterials 20:1167-1175, 1999.
118. Ye Q, Zund G, Benedikt P, Jockenhoevel S, Hoerstrup SP, Sakyama S, Hubbell JA, Turina M. Fibrin gel as a three dimensional matrix in cardiovascular tissue engineering. Eur J Cardiothorac Surg 17:587-591, 2000.
119. Tholpady SS, Schlosser R, Spotnitz W, Ogle RC, Lindsey WH. Repair of an osseous facial critical-size defect using augmented fibrin sealant. Laryngoscope 109:1585-1588, 1999.
120. Wechselberger G, Russell RC, Neumeister MW, Schoeller T, Piza-Katzer H, Rainer C. Successful transplantation of three tissue-engineered cell types using capsule induction technique and fibrin glue as a delivery vehicle. Plast Reconstr Surg 110:123-129, 2002.
121. Martinez J, Ferber A, Bach TL, Yaen CH. Interaction of fibrin with VE-cadherin. Ann N Y Acad Sci 936:386-405, 2001.
122. Cole M, Cox S, Mogford J, Mana M, Ho W, Eggleston A, Mustoe T, Tawil N. Fibrin sealant Tisseel is a biocompatible polymer for human-derived monocytes, fibroblasts and keratinocytes. Oral presentation—The Wound Healing Society, 11th Annual Conference, Albuquerque, NM, 2001.
123. Cox S, Mogford J, Cole M, Mustoe T, Tawil N. Fibrin sealant is an excellent biologic polymer for cell delivery: Fibroblasts–fibrin sealant construct for treating chronic wounds: In vitro and in vivo studies. Oral presentation, Society for Biomaterials, Tampa, Fla, 2002.

124. Ho W, Catelas I, Sese N, Cole M, Tawil B. Mesenchymal stem cell behavior in fibrin sealant: In vitro studies. Oral presentation—29th Annual Meeting Society for Biomaterials, Reno, Nev, 2003.
125. Ferguson R, Cox S, Sese N, Cole M, Tawil B. The use of fibrin sealant to deliver neuronal stem cell: In vitro studies. Oral presentation—29th Annual Meeting Society of Biomaterials, Reno, Nev, 2003.
126. Sese N, Cole M, Cox S, Tawil N. Delivering human keratinocytes using fibrin sealant: In vitro studies. Oral presentation—13th Annual Conference of the Wound Healing Society, Seattle, Wash, 2003.
127. Cox S, Cole M, Tawil N. The behavior of human dermal fibroblasts in 3 dimensional fibrin clots: Dependence on the fibrinogen, fibronectin and thrombin concentration (in press).
128. Lippert H, Wolff H. Erfahrungen mit fibrinkleberbeschichteten Kollagenvlies. [Experiences with fibrin glue–coated collagen fleece]. Zentralbl Chir 115:1175-1180, 1990.
129. Harris P, Capperauld I. Clinical experience in neurosurgery with absele: A new absorbable haemostatic bone sealant. Surg Neurol 13:231-235, 1980.
130. Jackson MR, Taher MM, Burge JR, Krishnamurti C, Reid TJ, Alving BM. Hemostatic efficacy of a fibrin sealant dressing in an animal model of kidney injury. J Trauma 45: 662-665, 1998.
131. Prior JJ, Wallace DG, Harner A, Powers N. A sprayable hemostat containing fibrillar collagen, bovine thrombin, and autologous plasma. Ann Thorac Surg 68:479-485, 1999.
132. Oz MC, Cosgrove DM III, Badduke BR, Hill JD, Flannery MR, Palumbo R, Topic N. Controlled clinical trial of a novel hemostatic agent in cardiac surgery. The Fusion Matrix Study Group. Ann Thorac Surg 69:1376-1382, 2000.
133. Bachet J, Goudot B, Teodori G, Brodaty D, Dubois C, De Lentdecker P, Guilmet D. Surgery of type A acute aortic dissection with Gelatine-Resorcine-Formol biological glue: A twelve-year experience. J Cardiovasc Surg (Torino) 31:263-273, 1990.
134. Portoghese M, Acar C, Jebara V, Chachques JC, Fontaliran F, Deloche A, Carpentier A. Changes in the vascular wall induced by surgical glues. Experimental study. Presse Med 21:1154-1156, 1992.
135. Erasmi AW, Sievers HH, Wolschlager C. Inflammatory response after BioGlue application. Ann Thorac Surg 73:1025-1026, 2002.
136. Fabiani JN, Jebara VA, Deloche A, Stephan Y, Carpentier A. Use of surgical glue without replacement in the treatment of type A aortic dissection. Circulation 80:I264-I268, 1989.
137. Ellis DA, Shaikh A. The ideal tissue adhesive in facial plastic and reconstructive surgery. J Otolaryngol 19:68-72, 1990.
138. Coover H, Joyner, Shearer N, et al. Chemistry performance of cyanoacrylate adhesives. J Surg Res 15:5-6, 1959.
139. Watson DR, Maguda TA. An experimental study for closure of tympanic membrane perforations with fascia and an adhesive. South Med J 58:844-847, 1965.
140. Toriumi DM, Taslan WF, Friedman M, Tardy ME. Histotoxicity of cyanoacrylate tissue adhesives: A comparison study. Arch Otorhinolaryngol Head Neck Surg 116:545-550, 1990.
141. Samson D, Marshall D. Carcinogenic potential of isobutyl-2-cyanoacrylate. J Neurosurg 65:571-572, 1986.
142. Cavanaugh TB, Gottsch JD. Infectious keratitis and cyanoacrylate adhesive. Am J Ophthalmol 111:466-472, 1991.
143. Waite JH. The formation of mussel byssus: Anatomy of a natural manufacturing process. In Case ST, ed. Structure, Cellular Synthesis and Assembly of Biopolymers. New York: Springer-Verlag, 1992.
144. Laursen RA. Reflection on the structure of mussel adhesive protein. In Case ST, ed. Structure, Cellular Synthesis and Asssembly of Biopolymers. New York: Springer-Verlag, 1992.

145. Pitman MI, Menche D, Song EK, Ben Yishay A, Gilbert D, Grande DA. The use of adhesives in chondrocyte transplantation surgery: In-vivo studies. Bull Hosp Jt Dis Orthop Inst 49:213-220, 1989.
146. Fulkerson JP, Norton LA, Gronowicz G, Picciano P, Massicotte JM, Nissen CW. Attachment of epiphyseal cartilage cells and 17/28 rat osteosarcoma osteoblasts using mussel adhesive protein. J Orthop Res 8:793-798, 1990.
147. Liggett PE, Cano M, Robin JB, Green RL, Lean JS. Intravitreal biocompatibility of mussel adhesive protein. A preliminary study. Retina 10:144-147, 1990.
148. Hill A, Estridge TD, Maroney M, Monnet E, Egbert B, Cruise G, Coker GT. Treatment of suture line bleeding with a novel synthetic surgical sealant in a canine iliac PTFE graft model. J Biomed Mater Res 58:308-312, 2001.
149. FDA talk paper. www.fda.gov/bbs/topics/ANSWERS/ANS01018 html 2003.
150. Kobayashi H, Sekine T, Nakamura T, Shimizu Y. In vivo evaluation of a new sealant material on a rat lung air leak model. J Biomed Mater Res 58:658-665, 2001.

CHAPTER

2

Tissue Sealants Available Today

Martin J. MacPhee, Ph.D. ▪ Belinda K. Wilmer, M.S.

The purpose of this chapter is to provide the history and forms of surgical sealants, followed by a detailed survey of the available products, their uses, and the considerations that may influence their use.

The use of sealants in surgery dates to at least the Egyptian Empire[1] and possibly earlier. Beginning with pioneering efforts to use polymerized fibrin clots as a hemostatic agent in World War I,[2] the twentieth century witnessed an expansion in both the number and capabilities of these useful surgical tools. Following World War I, the purification of thrombin by Seeger[2] paved the way for the development of the first fibrin sealant by Cronkite and Tidrick in 1940.[3] In 1941 these innovations were developed into commercial products (Fig. 2-1) that were fielded in the United States for several years until concerns about viral transmission resulted in their being withdrawn from the market in the 1950s. The contemporaneous development of cyanoacrylate adhesives led to their use as hemostatic tools in the Vietnam War, but again, postwar concerns over safety kept these products off the domestic market.[4]

Fibrin sealants were largely forgotten until their rediscovery in the 1970s, when production of second-generation fibrin sealants boasted measures to improve viral safety that resulted in their licensure in Europe and Canada in the 1970s and 1980s.[5] Confusion at the U.S. Food and Drug Administration (FDA) regarding their efficacy kept these products off the market in the United States. A conference on surgical sealants in 1993 demonstrated (First International Symposium on Surgical Adhesives) the potential for these products within the community of U.S. researchers, regulators, and clinicians working with these surgical tools. In 1993 the senior author (M.J.M.) and others urged the U.S. Army Medical Command to confront the FDA with these issues, and the result was a consensus conference, held in Bethesda, Md., in 1994, that made the need for these products clear to the FDA.[6] Subsequent conferences on surgical sealants chaired by M.J.M. and held by the Cambridge Healthtech Institute from 1996 to 2002 further elucidated the need for fibrin sealant products and the opportunities for other surgical sealants to increase the therapeutic options available to surgeons. As a result of this educational process, the FDA changed its require-

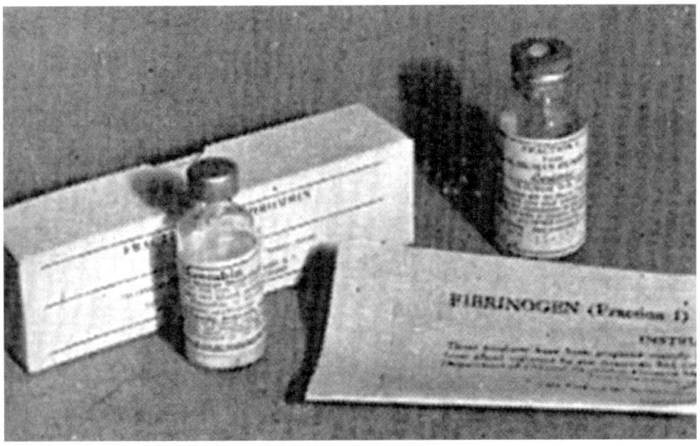

Figure 2-1 The first fibrin sealant product—Human Fibrinogen and Thrombin Kit—was produced in the United States during World War II. (From Andrus E, Bronk D, Carden G Jr, Keefer C, Lockwood J, Wearn J, eds. Advances in Military Medicine, vol. 1. Boston: Little, Brown, 1948.)

ments for licensure of fibrin sealants in 1997, and in 1998 a commercial fibrin sealant product was again available in the United States.[7] Licensure of the first cyanoacrylate product for human use followed shortly, and in the past 5 years more than 15 tissue sealant/gluing products, representing over a dozen distinct chemistries, have been registered for use in the United States.

Throughout this process, cosmetic and reconstructive surgical needs have been a significant driver for the development and use of these products. One of the first applications for a fibrin sealant based on plasma and thrombin was nerve anastomosis,[2] and the first large-scale use of fibrin sealants was in skin grafting of burn victims in World War II, beginning in 1941.[3] Subsequently it was a plastic surgeon who rediscovered these products and urged their development in Europe.[8] Plastic and reconstructive surgeons contributed significantly to the continuing pressure put on the FDA during the 1990s that resulted in the relicensure of fibrin sealants in the United States. Furthermore, the first of the cyanoacrylate products was registered in the United States for a cosmetic application.[4]

In this chapter we will describe the various types of surgical sealants available in the United States today. The safety and efficacy of each will be examined, and their uses described with particular emphasis on their applications in cosmetic and reconstructive surgery.

These products may be defined in many ways, the simplest being by their intended uses, which are broadly characterized as hemostasis and sealing/gluing. Of these, hemostasis has the longest modern history, and a large number of

TABLE 2-1 CONTEMPORARY HEMOSTATIC TISSUE GLUE PRODUCTS

Product Type	Constituents	Examples
Fibrin sealant: Pooled	Fibrinogen and thrombin (human) + Tranexamic acid	Crosseal
	Fibrinogen and thrombin (human) + Aprotinin	Hemaseel APR, Tisseel VH
Fibrin sealant: Autologous*	Fibrinogen and thrombin (human) and Bovine thrombin	Autoseal
Platelet gels*	Autologous platelets and bovine thrombin	SmartPReP2 *APC*$^{+}$, Magellan
Collagen-based: Autologous	Autologous plasma and bovine collagen and bovine thrombin	CoStasis
Collagen-based: Bovine	Microcrystalline bovine collagen	Avitene
Gelatin-based	Bovine gelatin and bovine thrombin	FloSeal
Synthetic hydrogel	Polyethylene glycol polymer (PEG)	CoSeal

*Device for producing.

TABLE 2-2 SEALING TISSUE GLUE PRODUCTS

Product Type	Constituents	Examples
Fibrin sealant: Pooled	Fibrinogen and thrombin (human)	Crosseal
	Fibrinogen and thrombin (human) + Aprotinin	Hemaseel APR, Tisseel VH
Fibrin sealant: Autologous*	Fibrinogen and thrombin (human) and bovine thrombin	Autoseal
Platelet gels*	Autologous platelets and bovine thrombin	SmartPReP2 *APC*$^{+}$, Magellan
Cyanoacrylate	Methyl-ethyl-cyanoacrylate†	Krazy Glue
	(Iso)(n)butyl-cyanoacrylate	Indermil, Trufill, Liquid Bandage, Vetbond‡
	Octyl-cyanoacrylate	Dermabond, Orabase Soothe-N-Seal, BAND-AID, Liquid Bandage, Nexaband‡
Synthetic hydrogel	Polyethylene glycol polymer (PEG)	CoSeal
Photopolymerized synthetic hydrogel	Primer, sealant (PEG polymer), and light wand	FocalSeal-L
Albumin-glutaraldehyde	Bovine albumin and glutaraldehyde	BioGlue

*Device for producing.
†Not to be used in medical applications because of local toxicity. Included for information purposes only.
‡Product approved for veterinary use.

these hemostatic products are currently registered in the United States. Although many of these products are currently licensed for relatively limited applications, the reality is that they are broadly used in medical practice for control of mild-to-moderate bleeding, often in an off-label manner. Table 2-1 shows a partial list of such products currently approved for clinical use in the United States.

Table 2-2 lists those products that are used primarily for their sealing capability. Several products appear in both tables, evidence of the closely related nature of these applications. Yet it is also significant that as many products also appear in only one of these tables and that these are generally the most modern products, with (semi)artificial chemistries that are more single purpose in their activity than, for example, fibrinogen, which is engineered by nature to serve both functions. In the discussions that follow, we will examine all of these products within their respective classes and individually.

Fibrin Sealants

The modern history of surgical sealants has been largely driven by the discovery, rediscovery, and refinement of the fibrin sealant technology. These products are sometimes referred to as fibrin glues, although in the past decade the term "fibrin sealant" has gained favor, as it more accurately conveys the hemostatic and tissue-sealing capabilities of the product; the term "glue" is afforded to other compounds that have greater tensile strength.

Fibrin sealing initially was invented by Cronkite et al.[2,3]; the first commercial fibrin sealant products were developed in the United States during World War II. Originally consisting of animal thrombin and human fibrinogen derived from pooled human plasma, the products were refined into an "all human" product, which eventually was withdrawn from the market because of hepatitis transmission by the thrombin component.[5] Decades later the technology was rediscovered in Europe, and the first European product, which was manufactured with improved antiviral processing steps, debuted in 1976 in Austria.[9] Interestingly, this was also a combination human-animal product, containing both bovine thrombin and aprotinin.[5] The bovine thrombin eventually was replaced by human thrombin, although the bovine aprotinin remains in the product licensed in the United States. Its use is controversial, as there is no clinical data supporting its benefit except in surgery on certain patients with hemophilia,[10-13] and preclinical studies comparing it to aprotinin-free fibrin sealant are equivocal. Generally in vitro and in vivo studies in which only clot recovery has been studied tend to show an increased clot retention afforded by antifibrinolytics,[7,14] whereas in vivo surgical models that quantify hemostatic performance have shown no difference.[15] Several more modern fibrin sealants that do not contain aprotinin or other antifibrinolytics have been shown to be as effective or more effective than the licensed product in both preclinical and clinical studies.[15-18]

Currently three products are available in the United States. Two are identical products manufactured by Baxter-Immuno AG (Vienna, Austria) and sold as Tisseel and Hemaseel APR by Baxter Corporation (Deerfield, Ill.) and Haemacure Corporation (Montreal, Quebec, Canada), respectively. The third, Crosseal, is manufactured by Omrix Biopharmaceuticals, Ltd. (Belgium) for the American Red Cross; it recently was approved by the FDA and is expected to reach the marketplace shortly.[19] Although Tisseel and Hemaseel APR contain bovine aprotinin, Crosseal does not.[20] A version of this product sold in Europe contained tranexamic acid in place of aprotinin.[7] Following several deaths associated with its use in neurosurgery and the discovery that tranexamic acid was neurotoxic,[21] the product was relabeled with a warning against its use in neurologic or spinal procedures. Crosseal carries a warning that it must not be brought in contact with cerebrospinal fluid or dura mater.[20]

Fibrin sealants may also be produced in another form in which the fibrinogen component is derived from the blood of a single donor. This single-donor material may be either heterologous or autologous with respect to the recipient, with the latter being most favored for its perceived safety value, although this has been questioned.[7] Originally produced in blood banks using general laboratory equipment, these so-called home-brew sealants had a reputation for spotty performance, associated with a low and highly variable level of clottable protein (fibrinogen). The availability of special machines designed to manufacture the fibrinogen component offers the possibility of more reliable product performance.[8,22-25] The CryoSeal FS system (Thermogenesis Corp., Rancho Cordova, Calif.)—a machine plus disposables system capable of generating multiple doses of both the fibrinogen and thrombin components of single-donor fibrin sealant—is licensed overseas and currently is in late phase III evaluation in the United States[26] (MacPhee M., personal communication, 2003). Although current statistics are unavailable, it is interesting to note that despite the perceived advantages of autologous and blood bank–derived fibrin sealants over commercial products, by 2001 commercial fibrin sealants outsold home-brew sealants 3 to 1 at a large hospital system with a considerable commitment to tissue sealant technology.[27]

Another related type of sealant is platelet gel. These gels typically are produced in a manner quite similar to single-donor fibrin sealant, which uses machines designed for this purpose (see Table 2-1). Although claims are made that these gels achieve a result superior to that of some fibrin sealants, their overall benefit is unclear. These results usually are attributed to growth factors released from platelets upon their activation by thrombin; however, so far this means of wound closure does not represent a significant component of surgical sealant use, making its relative value difficult to ascertain. Previously these home-brew products also have suffered from variable concentration issues; however, automated production devices now available largely eliminate this issue.[8,22-25] The gels' continuing reliance on bovine thrombin carries with it the same risks as will be described for single-donor fibrin sealant.

Safety

Pooled fibrin sealants have an enviable track record of safety. With the previously described exceptions, their proper use has not been associated with known fatalities. Since the development of the second-generation products in the 1970s, the only reported instances of disease transmission have been of human parvovirus B19.[28] This produces a generally benign infection in patients, with at most a transient alteration in red blood cell counts and mild fever, corresponding to the disease it is known to cause in children, fifth disease. The number of adverse events of all types that have been reported is low as compared to what is reported to be millions of treatments worldwide[7] but may be higher than suspected for some preparations.[29] A single case of HIV transmission has also been alleged.[30] Newer sealants in development incorporate more advanced viral inactivation and removal steps that should further decrease the already small risk of viral transmission. There remain concerns regarding the inclusion of the bovine component aprotinin. Antibody responses, including both IgG and IgE, have been observed following exposure to this protein via fibrin sealant,[31-33] and care should be given to minimize its use, particularly in patients with a history of prior exposure.[31] With the continuing spread of bovine spongiform encephalopathy (BSE) and other animal prion diseases to countries previously believed to be "free" of these agents, the potential for transmission to patients should be considered. Overall these risks are small, as evidenced by the 25-year history of these second-generation fibrin sealants. Robust viral inactivation and removal steps used during processing should minimize the risks of exposure to emerging viral threats such as West Nile virus[34] and the occasional adventitious agent such as Monkeypox.

There is no clear evidence regarding the safety of home-brew products, but it seems reasonable to assume that single-donor, nonautologous materials carry a risk of infection by known agents of concern similar to that of blood components, which is approximately 1 in 1 million with appropriate nucleic acid testing of donors. Viruses not tested for will not be eliminated in processing, as these products, in contrast to pooled products, employ no pathogen inactivation or removal steps, possibly reducing their perceived safety advantage.[7] There is a single report of a case of HIV-1 transmission associated with nonautologous single-donor fibrin sealant.[30,33] The risks associated with autologous processing are not quantified, but include improper processing, handling, and storage, as well as the risk of a clerical error that allows a product made from the blood of one patient to be used in another. To date, these risks also appear quite low as there are no reports of adverse events stemming from such occurrences.

A more compelling risk associated with the use of single-donor fibrin sealant is the exposure to bovine thrombin. This biological, previously believed to be benign, was shown to be the cause of both fatal and nonfatal coagulopathies associated with both direct injection into the circulation and use as a topical hemostat.[35] The rapid-onset disseminated coagulation associated with inadvertent direct injection of thrombin, although at first thought to be an inherent property of thrombin, was later demonstrated to be associated with impurities within the bovine preparations then in use.[36] Similar problems were not seen with highly purified human thrombin characteristic of third-generation pooled fibrin sealants.[36] The development of a hemorrhagic diathesis following exposure to bovine thrombin was likewise found to be a result of an antibody response to bovine coagulation factor V contaminants within the thrombin preparation that cross-reacted with the patient's own factor V.[27,37,38] These reactions ranged from benign to severe. Collectively these concerns led to the voluntary withdrawal of the least pure bovine thrombin products from the market, although the safety profile of the remaining products is not fully characterized. Finally, just as for pooled products employing bovine aprotinin, the exposure to bovine components represents a small hazard due to the risk of prion transmission. Single-donor preparations containing bovine thrombin should be used in light of these as yet uncharacterized risks.

Efficacy

Fibrin sealants have been shown to be efficacious in every organ system and surgical specialty. They have two main and several additional uses. Their principal uses are for hemostasis and sealing/adhesion. They have been demonstrated to be effective at stopping otherwise difficult to control oozing and frank hemorrhage from such disparate tissue as bone,[7] vascular anastomoses[7,8,39] and splenic and hepatic trauma.[40] Fibrin sealants frequently have been shown to prevent or reduce ecchymosis following cosmetic and reconstructive surgeries.[41,42] Most applications for cosmetic surgery have been successful using either pooled or autologous fibrin sealants. Experimental forms have even demonstrated the ability to halt otherwise fatal hemorrhage due to traumatic injury of the liver[43] or extremities[44] and currently are undergoing clinical trials.

The use of fibrin sealants for sealing/adhesion applications is similarly broad based and compelling. Fibrin sealants have been used to control air leaks,[8] urine leakage,[45] cerebrospinal fluid leakage in numerous neurologic reconstructive procedures,[4,46] and lymphatic leakage following head and neck resection.[4,47,48] They also have been shown to be effective at reducing seroma formation in animal models[49] and drainage volume and time following clinical mastectomy and axillary resection when proper application technique is employed.[50,51] They have been similarly useful in reducing seroma formation and ecchymosis in cosmetic procedures including blepharoplasty and rhytidectomy.[23,22] Fibrin sealants were shown to be a valuable tool in nerve grafting as early as World War II,[2,52] and they continue in this role today.[53-58] They are also a useful adjunct to skin grafting procedures, where they have been shown to decrease seromas,[49] increase graft take,[23,41] and permit the use of sheet grafts on difficult sites such as the hand, affording earlier onset of rehabilitation and improved cosmesis.[59] Fibrin sealant also has been used as an adjunct to the treatment of pressure sores.[60] In many of these situations the fibrin sealant is filling a multifunctional role by controlling hemorrhage and serous leakage by sealing blood vessels, lymphatics, and tissue tracts while simultaneously assisting in the adherence of grafted structures. Platelet gels have been used similarly for numerous cosmetic surgical applications including mastopexy, breast augmentation, rhytidectomy, and neck lifts,[22,23] and for oral and maxillofacial procedures.[25] To date the claims that wound healing with platelet gels is superior to that with pooled fibrin sealant products remain undemonstrated. Regardless, platelet gels are certainly acceptable alternatives to pooled fibrin sealants in certain circumstances, that is, when the logistical temporal and quality control burdens associated with their preparations and the legal liability issues attending their manufacture by health care practitioners are justified. These same issues have virtually eliminated the use of single-donor fibrin sealants at one of the busiest tissue sealant–oriented surgical institutions.[27]

In most cases the application of fibrin sealants for hemorrhage control alone is simple and straightforward, with the major training issues revolving around the preparation of the material and the necessity for a largely dry field free of brisk bleeding. It should be noted that some investigators have questioned the suitability of the available hemostatic pooled formulations for sealing applications, noting that the high thrombin concentrations they contain result in a rapid setting that makes appropriate tissue apposition difficult.[61] There is experimental evidence that these high concentrations (1000 NIH U/ml) may compromise flap take by inducing microvascular thrombosis.[62] This was not seen with lower concentrations of thrombin and may not be expected to occur in purer human thrombin preparations. It should be noted that this phenomenon has not been a noted issue in clinical studies. Sealing applications often require more care, as it is possible to apply the material incorrectly, resulting in a barrier to wound healing.[61] An example is the use of fibrin sealants in mastectomy repair. Conflicting reports showing efficacy[50,51] and a lack of efficacy[63] can be attributed to the use of inappropriate technique. Most frequently this is related to the relationship between the setting time of the sealant and the time between application and bringing together the surfaces to be sealed. Most hemostatic formulations are designed to set quickly. When these formulations are applied for sealing, the surgeon must plan carefully to be able to bring the tissue faces together without gaps before the sealant sets. The use of a lower concentration of thrombin is advisable for these applications.[64] To achieve a successful outcome, surgeons should seek training and appropriate education, which are the goals of this volume.

Cyanoacrylates

Originally discovered in the 1940s by Eastman Kodak, cyanoacrylates are adhesive compounds characterized by their polymerization, in the presence of water, into a glue with high tensile and adhesive strengths. They are characterized according to the length of the carbon chain conjugated to the cyanoacrylate component. The original products were methyl- and ethyl-cyanoacrylate. The first generation of these strong adhesives was used in the Vietnam War and was submitted to the FDA in 1964.[65,66] Original reports were positive; however, these glues were essentially permanent, and foreign body reactions could be severe. This, along with concerns regarding their long-term toxicity and possible carcinogenicity, led to the development of a less permanent, more resorbable alternative. Researchers learned that by lengthening the carbon chains, they created adhesives of comparable strength but with less reactivity. An array of products aimed at the consumer and veterinary and medical marketplaces have been introduced. With their shortened regulatory pathways, the veterinary products were the first to debut. Vetbond and Nexaband, isobutyl- and octyl-cyanoacrylate, respectively, were the first such products available in the United States and, despite their labeling, have seen occasional use in human patients. The corresponding human products, Indermil (United States Surgical, Norwalk, Conn.), Trufill (Cordis Neurovascular, Inc., Miami Lakes, Fla.), and Dermabond (Ethicon, Somerville, N.J.), are more appropriate for this use. Trufill is intended for use as a sclerosing agent.[4,67] Dermabond, in contrast, is licensed for final closure of superficial wounds, particularly facial and scalp lacerations.[4] Whether used alone for superficial lacerations or in concert with deeper suture support, these adhesives permit a sutureless closure. This may be particularly desirable for facial injuries and in the treatment of children.[68,69] Cyanoacrylates have also been employed for other cosmetic applications, including blepharoplasty,[70,71] and even for full-thickness skin grafting.[72] Butyl-2-cyanoacrylate available in the United Kingdom has been reported to be a suitable means of closure for endaural incisions[73] and, with some limitations, for craniofacial fixation of structures with small loading levels.[24,70,74] Some studies have reported superior cosmetic outcomes for incisional wounds of adolescents closed with sutures rather than with Dermabond,[75] suggesting that further clinical research may continue to refine the decision-making process for selecting optimal means of wound closure. Nevertheless, cyanoacrylates are clearly an effective and appropriate choice for a wide range of wound closure challenges. The scope of their application has even expanded to include their use on recently deceased patients.[76]

Collagen and Gelatin-Based Products

Collagen and its denatured counterpart, gelatin, have a long history as topical hemostatic agents that began during World War II.[2] Gelatin sponges are still in use today, and more advanced forms of these hemostatic agents are increasing the choices available for surgical hemostasis. Microcrystalline collagen (Avitene, Davol Inc., Cranston, R.I.) can be used to control slow oozing. A recently available hemostatic product about which little is known is a fibrillar collagen from Collagen Matrix, Inc. The formulations of bovine thrombin and gelatin (FloSeal, Baxter Corporation, Deerfield, Ill.) or collagen plus autologous plasma (CoStasis, Cohesion Technologies, Inc., Palo Alto, Calif.) are generally more effective hemostatic preparations than collagen alone. Although generally less hemostatically powerful than pooled fibrin sealants,[39] these products have been shown to be active at controlling hemorrhages, particularly for vascular surgery,[77,78] and as sealants to control cerebrospinal fluid leaks.[79] The appropriate use for these sealants in cosmetic procedures is less clear, as they have been available for only a short time. The perception that collagen may persist at the site of application obviously raises questions; however, some of these products are known to resorb and so may produce acceptable cosmetic results.

Albumin-Based Products

For many years, European surgeons have used a group of powerful adhesives that contain a soluble protein component coupled with a nonspecific cross-linking agent such as glutaraldehyde, formalin, or resorcinol.[8] A commercial product utilizing bovine albumin and glutaraldehyde has been registered in the United States (BioGlue, CryoLife Inc., Kennesaw, Ga.). This product has great tensile strength and is tolerant of changes to the underlying tissue structure. It is intended for such applications as the treatment of dissecting abdominal aneurysms.[4] At this time, albumin-based products appear to have no role in cosmetic surgery, although their potential in this arena is unexplored.

Synthetic Hydrogels

Several surgical sealants have been developed that involve the use of synthetic polymer hydrogels. One of these is a polyethylene glycol (PEG)–based polymer system (CoSeal, Cohesion Technologies, Inc.). CoSeal has been used for hemostatic applications in vascular surgery.[80-82] CoSeal has also been tested in an animal model and found to prevent the formation of cardiac adhesions.[83] The second member of this group of sealants is a photopolymerized PEG polymer hydrogel that has been shown to be useful in treating experimental vascular[84] and reinforced intestinal anastomoses.[85] It is a light-cured PEG polymer that requires the application of a priming solution to the tissue surface to be treated. This product (FocalSeal-L, Genzyme Biosurgery, Cambridge, Mass.) has been used both experimentally and clinically to seal postoperative air leaks.[85] As is true for the albumin-based products, these recently available materials have not been evaluated for their utility in cosmetic procedures.

Conclusion

Beginning with the introduction of the first fibrin sealant in the 1940s, interest in the use of surgical sealants has grown. This interest has fueled the development of an expanding array of surgical tools. The registration of commercial, readily available tools, somewhat halting at first, has in time resulted in an impressive array of experimental and clinical studies supporting the use of these products in cosmetic and reconstructive surgery. Already in use for procedures ranging from embryo implantation[86] to postmortem cryopreservation,[76] these versatile surgical tools have applications that literally extend from before the cradle to past the grave. As more novel materials and applications become available, the impact of surgical sealants upon the ease and outcome of cosmetic procedures can only be expected to continue to grow in scope and significance.

REFERENCES

1. Sierra D. Fibrin sealant adhesive systems: A review of their chemistry, material properties and clinical applications. Biomater Appl 7:309-352, 1993.
2. Andrus E, Bronk D, Carden G Jr, Keefer C, Lockwood J, Wearn J, eds. Advances in Military Medicine, vol 1. Boston: Little, Brown & Co, 1948.
3. Cohn EJ. The history of plasma fractionation. In Andrus E, Bronk D, Carden G Jr, Keefer C, Lockwood J, Wearn J, eds. Advances in Military Medicine, vol 1. Boston: Little, Brown & Co, 1948.
4. Reece TB, Maxey TS, Kron IL. A prospectus on tissue adhesives. Am J Surg 182:40S-44S, 2001.
5. MacPhee M. Commercial pooled fibrin sealant. In Saltz R, Sierra D, eds. Current Trends in Surgical Tissue Adhesives: Proceedings of the First International Symposium on Surgical Adhesives. Lancaster, Pa: Technomic Publishing Co, 1996.
6. Alving BM, Weinstein MJ, Finlayson JS, Menitove JE, Fratantoni JC. Fibrin sealant: Summary of a conference on characteristics and clinical uses. Transfusion 36:783-790, 1995.
7. Spotnitz WD. Commercial fibrin sealants in surgical care. Am J Surg 182:8S-14S, 2001.
8. Morikawa T. Tissue sealing. Am J Surg. 182:29S-35S, 2001.
9. Matras H, Dinges H, Manoli B. Zur Nahtlosen Interfaszikularen Nerventransplantation im Tierexperiment. Wien Med Wochenschr 122:517-523, 1972.
10. Martinowitz U, Varon D, Heim M. The role of fibrin tissue adhesives in surgery of haemophilia patients. Haemophilia 4:443-448, 1998.
11. Martinowitz U, Schulman S, Horoszowski H, Heim M. Role of fibrin sealants in surgical procedures on patients with hemostatic disorders. Clin Orthop 65-75, 1996.
12. Blinder D, Martinowitz U, Ardekian L, Peleg M, Taicher S. [Oral surgical procedures during anticoagulant therapy]. Harefuah 130:681-683, 727, 1996.
13. Tock B, Drohan W, Hess J, Pusateri A, Holcomb J, MacPhee M. Haemophilia and advanced fibrin sealant technologies. Haemophilia 4:449-455, 1998.
14. Pipan CM, Glasheen WP, Matthew TL, Gonias SL, Hwang LJ, Jane JA, Spotnitz WD. Effects of antifibrinolytic agents on the life span of fibrin sealant. J Surg Res 53:402-407, 1992.
15. Kheirabadi BS, Pearson R, Tuthill D, Rudnicka K, Holcomb JB, Drohan W, MacPhee MJ. Comparative study of the hemostatic efficacy of a new human fibrin sealant: Is an antifibrinolytic agent necessary? J Trauma 52:1107-1115, 2002.
16. Nervi C, Gamelli RL, Greenhalgh DG, Luterman A, Hansbrough JF, Achauer BM, Gomperts ED, Lee M, Navalta L, Cruciani TR. A multicenter clinical trial to evaluate the topical hemostatic efficacy of fibrin sealant in burn patients. J Burn Care Rehabil, 22:99-103, 2001.
17. Greenhalgh DG, Gamelli RL, Lee M, Delavari M, Lynch JB, Hansbrough JF, Achauer BM, Miller SF, MacPhee M, Bray GL. Multicenter trial to evaluate the safety and potential efficacy of pooled human fibrin sealant for the treatment of burn wounds. J Trauma 46:433-440, 1999.

18. McGill V, Kowal-Vern A, Lee M, Greenhalgh D, Gomperts E, Bray G, Gamelli R. Use of fibrin sealant in thermal injury. J Burn Care Rehabil 18:429-434, 1997.
19. U.S. Food and Drug Administration (FDA). Product Approval Letter. FDA Web Site 2003. 6-12-2003.
20. Crosseal Label. FDA Web Site 6-12-2003.
21. Schlag MG, Hopf R, Zifko U, Redl H. Epileptic seizures following cortical application of fibrin sealants containing tranexamic acid in rats. Acta Neurochir (Wien) 144:63-69, 2002.
22. Man D, Plosker H, Winland-Brown JE. The use of autologous platelet-rich plasma (platelet gel) and autologous platelet-poor plasma (fibrin glue) in cosmetic surgery. Plast Reconstr Surg 107:229-237, 2001.
23. Man D, Plosker H, Winland-Brown JE, Saltz R. Discussion: The use of autologous platelet-rich plasma (platelet gel) and autologous platelet-poor plasma (fibrin glue) in cosmetic surgery. Plast Reconstr Surg 107:238-239, 2001.
24. Gosain AK, Lyon VB. The current status of tissue glues: Part II. For adhesion of soft tissues. Plast Reconstr Surg 110:1581-1584, 2002.
25. Bhanot S, Alex JC. Current applications of platelet gels in facial plastic surgery. Facial Plast Surg 18:27-33, 2002.
26. Coehlo P. CryoSeal FS System U.S. Clinical Update, 2003.
27. Carroll JF, Moskowitz KA, Edwards NM, Hickey TJ, Rose EA, Budzynski AZ. Immunologic assessment of patients treated with bovine fibrin as a hemostatic agent. Thromb Haemost 76:925-931, 1996.
28. Hino M, Ishiko O, Honda KI, Yamane T, Ohta K, Takubo T, Tatsumi N. Transmission of symptomatic parvovirus B19 infection by fibrin sealant used during surgery. Br J Haematol 108:194-195, 2000.
29. Kawamura M, Sawafuji M, Watanabe M, Horinouchi H, Kobayashi K. Frequency of transmission of human parvovirus B19 infection by fibrin sealant used during thoracic surgery. Ann Thorac Surg 73:1098-1100, 2002.
30. Wilson S, Pell P, Donegan E. HIV-1 transmission following the use of cryoprecipitated fibrinogen as gel adhesive. Transfusion 31:51, 1991.
31. Beierlein W, Scheule AM, Antoniadis G, Braun C, Schosser R. An immediate, allergic skin reaction to aprotinin after reexposure to fibrin sealant. Transfusion 40:302-305, 2000.
32. Scheule AM, Beierlein W, Wendel HP, Eckstein FS, Heinemann MK, Ziemer G. Fibrin sealant, aprotinin, and immune response in children undergoing operations for congenital heart disease. J Thorac Cardiovasc Surg 115:883-889, 1998.
33. Scheule AM, Beierlein W, Wendel HP, Jurmann MJ, Eckstein FS, Ziemer G. Aprotinin in fibrin tissue adhesives induces specific antibody response and increases antibody response of high-dose intravenous application. J Thorac Cardiovasc Surg 118:348-353, 1999.
34. AABB. Statement of the American Association of Blood Banks, America's Blood Centers, and the American Red Cross: Voluntary withdrawal of frozen blood products to mitigate risk of transmission of west Nile virus. AABB Web Site 12-12-2002.
35. Berguer R, Staerkel RL, Moore EE, Moore FA, Galloway WB, Mockus MB. Warning: Fatal reaction to the use of fibrin glue in deep hepatic wounds. Case reports. J Trauma 31:408-411, 1991.
36. Pusateri A, Holcomb J, Harris R, Gomez R, Hetz S, Enriquez J, Hess J. Hemodynamic effect of intravenous bovine or human thrombin in swine. Abstract presented at the Sixteenth Congress of the International Society on Thrombosis and Haemostasis, Florence, Italy, 1997. Thromb Haemost Suppl 1997.
37. Muntean W, Zenz W, Finding K, Zobel G, Beitzke A. Inhibitor to factor V after exposure to fibrin sealant during cardiac surgery in a two-year-old child. Acta Paediatr 83:84-87, 1994.

38. Streiff MB, Ness PM. Acquired FV inhibitors: A needless iatrogenic complication of bovine thrombin exposure. Transfusion 42:18-26, 2002.
39. Kheirabadi BS, Field-Ridley A, Pearson R, MacPhee M, Drohan W, Tuthill D. Comparative study of the efficacy of the common topical hemostatic agents with fibrin sealant in a rabbit aortic anastomosis model. J Surg Res 106:99-107, 2002.
40. Oschner MG, Maniscalco-Theberge ME, Champion HR. Fibrin glue as a hemostatic agent in hepatic and splenic trauma. Trauma 30:884-887, 1990.
41. Saltz R, Zamora S. Tissue adhesives and applications in plastic and reconstructive surgery. Aesthetic Plast Surg 22:439-443, 1998.
42. Ellis DA, Pelausa EO. Fibrin glue in facial plastic and reconstructive surgery. J Otolaryngol 17:74-77, 1988.
43. Holcomb JB, Pusateri AE, Hess JR, Hetz SP, Harris RA, Tock BB, Drohan WN, MacPhee MJ. Implications of new dry fibrin sealant technology for trauma surgery. Surg Clin of North Am 77:943-952, 1997.
44. Hess J, Holcomb J, MacPhee M. Hemorrhage control with a dry powdered thrombin and fibrinogen bandage. Netherlands Defence Military Medical Review, 1996.
45. Pantanowitz L, Kruskall MS, Uhl L. Cryoprecipitate. Patterns of use. Am J Clin Pathol 119:874-881, 2003.
46. Ellis DA, Shaikh A. The ideal tissue adhesive in facial plastic and reconstructive surgery. J Otolaryngol 19:68-72, 1990.
47. Toriumi DM, Lovice D, O'Grady KM. Fibrin tissue adhesive in otolaryngology—head and neck surgery. J Long Term Eff Med Implants 8:143-159, 1998.
48. Toriumi DM, O'Grady K. Surgical tissue adhesives in otolaryngology—head and neck surgery. Otolaryngol Clin North Am 27:203-209, 1994.
49. Kulber DA, Bacilious N, Peters ED, Gayle LB, Hoffman L. The use of fibrin sealant in the prevention of seromas. Plast Reconstr Surg 99:842-849, 1997.
50. Moore MM, Freeman MG. 1998. Fibrin sealant in breast surgery. J Long Term Eff Med Implants 8:133-142.
51. Moore MM, Nguyen DH, Spotnitz WD. Fibrin sealant reduces serous drainage and allows for earlier drain removal after axillary dissection: A randomized prospective trial. Am Surg 63:97-102, 1997.
52. Work carried out between Office of Scientific Research and Development and Harvard University on products developed in the Department of Physical Chemistry, Harvard Medical School, from blood collected by the American Red Cross. In Clinical Uses of Products Made From Human Fibrinogen and Human Thrombin, 1943.
53. Wieken K, Angioi-Duprez K, Lim A, Marchal L, Merle M. Nerve anastomosis with glue: Comparative histologic study of fibrin and cyanoacrylate glue. J Reconstr Microsurg 19:17-20, 2003.
54. Bento RF, De Almeida ER, Miniti A. Anastomosis of intratemporal facial nerve with fibrin tissue adhesive. Eur Arch Otorhinolaryngol S387-S388, 1994.
55. Menovsky T, Bartels RH. Stabilization and accurate trimming of nerve ends: Practical use of fibrin glue: Technical note. Neurosurgery 44:224-225, 1999.
56. Egloff DV, Narakas A. Nerve anastomoses with human fibrin. Preliminary clinical report (56 cases). Ann Chir Main 2:101-115, 1983.
57. Bento RF, Miniti A. Anastomosis of the intratemporal facial nerve using fibrin tissue adhesive. Ear Nose Throat J 72:663, 1993.
58. Feldman MD, Sataloff RT, Epstein G, Ballas SK. Autologous fibrin tissue adhesive for peripheral nerve anastomosis. Arch Otolaryngol Head Neck Surg 113:963-967, 1987.
59. Saltz R, Sierra D, Feldman D, Bartczak-Saltz M, Dimick A, Vasconez LO. Experimental and clinical applications of fibrin glue. Plast Reconstr Surg 88:1005-1014, 1991.
60. Pers M, Snorrason K, Nielsen IM. Primary results following surgical treatment of pressure sores. Scand J Plast Reconstr Surg 20:123-124, 1986.

61. Forseth M, O'Grady K, Toriumi DM. The current status of cyanoacrylate and fibrin tissue adhesives. J Long Term Eff Med Implants 2:221-233, 1992.
62. Frost-Arner L, Spotnitz WD, Rodeheaver GT, Drake DB. Comparison of the thrombogenicity of internationally available fibrin sealants in an established microsurgical model. Plast Reconstr Surg 108:1655-1660, 2001.
63. Dinsmore RC, Harris JA, Gustafson RJ. Effect of fibrin glue on lymphatic drainage after modified radical mastectomy: A prospective randomized trial. Am Surg 66:982-985, 2000.
64. O'Grady KM, Agrawal A, Bhattacharyya TK, Shah A, Toriumi DM. An evaluation of fibrin tissue adhesive concentration and application thickness on skin graft survival. Laryngoscope 110:1931-1935, 2000.
65. Brock KV. The persistence of bovine viral diarrhea virus. Biologicals 31:133-135, 2003.
66. Frye A. Can we really use super glue instead of suture? Anne Frye electronic citation, 2003.
67. U.S. Food and Drug Administration (FDA). Trufill Approval Letter. FDA Web Site 7-10-2003.
68. Bruns TB, Worthington JM. Using tissue adhesive for wound repair: A practical guide to Dermabond. Am Fam Physician 61:1383-1388, 2000.
69. Craven NM, Telfer NR. An open study of tissue adhesive in full-thickness skin grafting. J Am Acad Dermatol 40:607-611, 1999.
70. Greene D, Koch RJ, Goode RL. Efficacy of octyl-2-cyanoacrylate tissue glue in blepharoplasty. A prospective controlled study of wound-healing characteristics. Arch Facial Plast Surg 1:292-296, 1999.
71. Shermak MA, Wong L, Inoue N, Chao EY, Manson PN. Butyl-2-cyanoacrylate fixation of mandibular osteotomies. Plast Reconstr Surg 102:319-324, 1998.
72. Quinn J, Wells G, Sutcliffe T, Jarmuske M, Maw J, Stiell I, Johns P. Tissue adhesive versus suture wound repair at 1 year: Randomized clinical trial correlating early, 3-month, and 1-year cosmetic outcome. Ann Emerg Med 32:645-649, 1998.
73. Bhalla RK, Lesser TH. Simple, painless, cosmetic closure of endaural incisions. J Laryngol Otol 117:67-68, 2003.
74. Amarante MT, Constantinescu MA, O'Connor D, Yaremchuk MJ. Cyanoacrylate fixation of the craniofacial skeleton: An experimental study. Plast Reconstr Surg 95:639-646, 1995.
75. Ong CC, Jacobsen AS, Joseph VT. Comparing wound closure using tissue glue versus subcuticular suture for pediatric surgical incisions: A prospective, randomized trial. Pediatr Surg Int 18:553-555, 2002.
76. Darwin M, Harris S, Russell S. Securing hemostasis in the human cryopreservation patient. BioPreservation, Inc. Electronic citation 1-25-1997.
77. CoStasis Multi-Center Collaborative Writing Committee. A novel collagen-based composite offers effective hemostatis for multiple surgical indications: Results of a randomized controlled trial. Surgery 129:445-450, 2001.
78. Oz MC, Cosgrove DM III, Badduke BR, Hill JD, Flannery MR, Palumbo R, Topic N. Controlled clinical trial of a novel hemostatic agent in cardiac surgery. The Fusion Matrix Study Group. Ann Thorac Surg 69:1376-1382, 2000.
79. Renkins KL, Payner TD, Leipzig TJ, Feuer H, Morone MA, Koers JM, Lawson KJ, Lentz R, Shuey H, Conaway GL, Andersson GBJ, An HS, Hickey M, Rondinone JF, Shargill NS. A multicenter, prospective, randomized trial evaluating a new hemostatic agent for spinal surgery. Spine 26:1645-1650, 2001.
80. Glickman M, Gheissari A, Money S, Martin J, Ballard JL. A polymeric sealant inhibits anastomotic suture hole bleeding more rapidly than gelfoam/thrombin: Results of a randomized controlled trial. Arch Surg 137:326-331, 2002.
81. Burger T, Gussman A, Krenzien J, Moll F, Coker G, Block J. Novel sealing agent inhibits suture-line bleeding in synthetic and autologous vascular grafts. European CoSeal Surgical Sealant Study Group, 2003.

82. Marc HM, Mees U, Hill AC, Egbert B, Coker GT, Estridge TD. Evaluation of a novel synthetic sealant for inhibition of cardiac adhesions and clinical experience in cardiac surgery procedures. Heart Surg. Forum 4:204-209, 2001.
83. Hill A, Estridge TD, Maroney M, Monnet E, Egbert B, Cruise G, Coker GT. Treatment of suture line bleeding with a novel synthetic surgical sealant in a canine iliac PTFE graft model. J Biomed Mater Res 58:308-312, 2001.
84. White JK, Titus JS, Tanabe H, Aretz T, Torchiana DF. The use of a novel tissue sealant as a hemostatic adjunct in cardiac surgery. Heart Surg Forum 3:56-61, 2000.
85. Sweeney T, Rayan S, Warren H, Rattner D. Intestinal anastomoses detected with a photopolymerized hydrogel. Surgery 131:185-189, 2002.
86. Ben Rafael Z, Ashkenazi J, Shelef M, Farhi J, Voliovitch I, Feldberg D, Orvieto R. The use of fibrin sealant in in vitro fertilization and embryo transfer. Int J Fertil Menopausal Stud 40:303-306, 1995.

CHAPTER

3

The Tissue Adhesive Decision: Algorithms for Successful Clinical Use

William D. Spotnitz, M.D. ▪ Sandra G. Burks, B.S.N.

Surgical Revolution

Miniaturization

The first tissue adhesive to be widely employed in the United States, fibrin sealant, initially was used in cardiac surgery as a hemostatic agent. Fibrin sealant was first approved in Europe in 1972, but it required almost a quarter of a century to pass the U.S. Food and Drug Administration (FDA) regulatory scrutiny for safety and effectiveness. Since fibrin sealant was approved in 1998, four other families of tissue adhesives have been approved, and this field is now rapidly advancing with the introduction of new and revised products. As with all modern technologies, the need for miniaturization is also affecting the specialty of surgery. Smaller instruments for microscopic tissue manipulation, robotics, and even cellular level procedures are becoming more and more common. In this environment tissue adhesives, which can help to minimize tissue trauma, are an extremely important modality. The five present families of tissue adhesives can achieve hemostasis, sealing, and tissue apposition. They can also be used for pneumostasis, lymphostasis, and vascular embolization.

Minimally Invasive Incisions

The future of surgery is closely related to more minimally invasive surgical approaches. Smaller incisions may be better tolerated by the patient and are cosmetically more appealing. The public is clearly excited by this opportunity, and as long as surgical results and outcomes remain excellent, more and more procedures will be performed through smaller and smaller "keyhole" incisions. An important caveat in this expanding minimally invasive trend is that outcomes not be adversely affected. The technical challenge of minimally invasive surgery is clear to every surgeon and requires higher levels of competence and training. The surgeon in almost every surgical specialty is now being faced with a need to perform more complex operative procedures through smaller incisions. At the same time surgeons are required to reduce costs, decrease the length of hospital stay, and improve outcomes by reducing morbidity and mortality. Thus the surgeon is facing an ever-increasing challenge in every specialty including cosmetic procedures.

Role of Tissue Adhesives

Any materials that can assist the surgeon in these increasingly challenging technical situations will be of value. The addition of tissue adhesives to the surgical armamentarium has given the operator a variety of new materials with powerful on-label uses and potentially even more significant off-label applications. In this chapter the on-label uses of each agent will be discussed under Approved Materials. Both the on- and off-label applications of the agents will be discussed under Clinical Algorithms. These new agents may result in safer procedures that may be achieved with reduced costs even when the expense of the tissue adhesive is included.

Tissue Adhesives

Evolution

Although surgeons had materials to make suture-like threads as early as the first century BC,[1] the use of glues in surgery is a relatively new concept.[1] Sutures are presently used to achieve tissue apposition and to control the leakage of blood, visceral fluids, lymph, and air. The use of sutures for these requirements has become a worldwide, multibillion-dollar industry. Just as sutures have become an indispensable weapon in the surgeon's armamentarium, tissue adhesives eventually may develop an equally important role. The analogy that can be used is that of the master cabinetmaker. This craftsman uses a saw to cut, nails to connect solid structures, and glue to keep more fragile objects together. The surgeon, however, has had a scalpel to cut, sutures to ensure strong tissue apposition, but no glues for more delicate applications. Thus the introduction of tissue adhesives should fulfill a significant need that is only being increased by the technologic challenges of minimally invasive surgery.

Ideal Adhesives

The ideal tissue adhesive should have strength in at least five significant areas.[2] First, the material needs to be safe. Neither the tissue adhesive itself nor its metabolic products should have any negative effects. There should be no allergic responses, no significant tissue fibrosis, and no possibility of disease transmission from bacteria, viruses, or other organisms, and the material should not be carcinogenic. Second, the agent needs to be effective. This is a complex issue, as effectiveness is different within each surgical specialty. A trauma surgeon wishing to achieve rapid hemostasis at the site of a penetrating injury will want a rapidly polymerizing strong adhesive with a significant hemostatic capacity. A cosmetic surgeon, on the other hand, may desire a more slowly polymerizing material that allows for arrangement of facial structures, flaps, or grafts. The cosmetic surgeon may need a material capable of eliminating potential spaces and decreasing tissue swelling and seroma formation. Clearly these characteristics are different. This suggests that multiple different forms of tissue adhesives may be required, just as there are different types of sutures: braided, monofilament, nonabsorbable, and absorbable are presently used. This need for multiple capabilities is not necessarily a deficiency in each individual tissue adhesive. Rather, materials may best meet these varied needs by being specifically engineered for a particular purpose. Thus it may be necessary to have multiple different tissue adhesives available in a given operating room, just as multiple different forms of sutures are currently available. Third, the material must be easily used. Usability should be evaluated in terms of the work required by surgical support personnel to prepare the agent as well as ease of application for the surgeon. The circulator or scrub nurse needs to be capable of rapidly reconstituting and preparing the material as well as loading the agent into whatever application tools have been devised. After these steps have been completed, the surgeon needs a material that can be easily and effectively applied in a variety of different settings. These include local pinpoint application or broad surface spraying. A surgeon should have accurate control with respect to the location of glue application, the thickness of application, and the rapidity of polymerization. Fourth, as with every new modality in our cost-conscious health care system, the use of tissue adhesives should decrease health care spending and improve the quality of results. Tissue adhesives should decrease operative costs even with the dollars required to buy the tissue adhesive itself included. Some of the new agents have a significant associated cost. However, some also have a dramatic clinical benefit that may justify their expense. Fifth, the material should meet the regulatory standards for safety and efficacy required for approval by the FDA for surgical tissue adhesives. Although this seems obvious, fibrin sealant, the first large-scale tissue adhesive approved for use in the United States, required almost a quarter of a century for approval by the FDA after it was initially licensed in 1972 in Europe. Thus facility in meeting FDA regulatory requirements is important, as the rapid introduction of safe and effective materials should be highly beneficial to surgeons, patients, and health care administrators.

Surgical Education

Although the application of surgical tissue adhesives would appear to be a relatively easily learned skill with almost trivial requirements for successful use, this is not the case. Just as the cabinetmaker needs to know the difference between various forms of synthetic adhesives and needs to skillfully and carefully place the glue, so the surgeon needs to know the characteristics of the various tissue adhesives and how to effectively apply them. In general, surgical education depends significantly on a period of apprenticeship in which the skills are developed in the young trainee over a period of several years. Technical skill increases as a surgeon learns to cut with both scalpel and scissors and to sew with a variety of different needle holders and forceps. Tissue adhesives, however, have only been recently introduced into the market. Thus most surgeons presently in practice have not had an opportunity to learn in depth the capacities of these new agents or how to properly apply them. In fact, the amount of time and effort spent in educating residents presently in training to use tissue adhesives is small compared to the time allotted for training in traditional surgical techniques. As the importance of the new tissue adhesive modalities increases, training in these techniques will increase in residency programs, and trainees will become more skilled in their use. For practicing physicians one of the most frequently used methods for learning new technologies is the visit from the commercial representative. Unfortunately these visits do not always offer hands-on experience and the careful technical instruction that is important in the use of these agents. More textbooks such as this one on cosmetic surgery as well as additional hands-on laboratory and clinical experience, may help to enhance the practicing physician's ability to effectively use these newly emerging materials.

Importance in Cosmetic Surgery

Improved Healing and Appearance

Although chapters in recent books have reviewed the field of tissue adhesives,[3-5] this is the first book devoted entirely to the use of these materials in cosmetic surgery. These agents have an important role to play in this field because they do help to reduce tissue trauma and can potentially enhance healing from surgical incisions. Some of the available agents, for example, fibrin sealant, are precursors of normal wound-healing processes and may be useful in accelerating wound healing by themselves. In the future, with the addition of appropriately engineered growth factors and medications, these adhesives may further accelerate the reparative process following surgical interventions. Because in selected situations these agents are less traumatic than suturing, less tissue injury may occur and wound appearance may be improved. This is particularly significant in facial cosmetic surgery, as early appearance and long-term results are critical. Anything that will improve early cosmesis and allow earlier resumption of normal activities as well as provide for an improved appearance over the long term is a beneficial intervention.

Less Swelling, Hematoma, and Ecchymosis

The available tissue adhesives have excellent ability to stop bleeding, seal lymphatics, eliminate potential spaces for serous fluid accumulation, and reduce tissue injury and destruction by eliminating the need for sutures. All these characteristics will significantly improve the appearance of wounds anywhere on the body. These new agents may reduce excessive tissue edema, hematoma formation, seroma accumulation, and ecchymosis. For example, blood vessels and lymphatics can be sealed at the same time that a skin flap is glued to the underlying muscle, thus avoiding the need for sutures. This decreases blood and lymphatic accumulation, reduces the potential space for seroma formation, and eliminates the need for sutures, which have the potential to cause further tissue injury. The new tissue adhesive modalities when properly used can substitute for sutures in specific settings and possibly result in wounds with an improved cosmetic appearance.

Approved Materials

Fibrin Sealant

Fibrin sealant was the first widely used tissue adhesive to be approved for use in the United States by the FDA. It consists of two major components: fibrinogen and thrombin, which in the presence of small amounts of factor XIII and calcium react to form polymerized fibrin, the final form of this biological tissue adhesive. The commercial product consists of human fibrinogen and thrombin that is derived from stores of pooled human plasma. Donors are prescreened using the traditional serologic techniques, and the pooled plasma products are virally inactivated with heat pasteurization and ultrafiltration. The concentration of fibrinogen in this product is 75 to 115 mg/ml, and the concentration of thrombin is 500 IU/ml. Bovine aprotinin is supplied in a concentration of 3000 KIU and is used as a stabilizer and antifibrinolytic agent. The aprotinin can reduce the rate of fibrinolysis associated with the use of fibrin sealant and thus reduce the rapidity of its biological degradation. Calcium is also provided in the commercial product; it is used as a catalyst in the reaction between fibrinogen and thrombin that forms fibrin sealant. Concerns about the safety of fibrin sealant are based mostly on the issue of possible disease transmission. Elimination of bacteria has been straightforward in this product, and aggressive measures are taken to reduce the possibility of viral disease transmission as well. Newer generations of product will add additional antiviral steps beyond the heat pasteurization and ultrafiltration presently provided. The risk of disease transmission beyond that of standard bacteria and viruses, such as prions, are unknown but thus far have not appeared clinically significant. Because the agent is biodegradable and is patterned along the normal mechanisms of the human clotting cascade, there is essentially no long-term risk of carcinogenicity. Initial reservations about potential fibrotic reactions at the site of fibrin sealant use have not been documented, and the material is almost completely biodegraded within a period of 2 to 4 weeks.

The FDA has approved fibrin sealant for two specific indications. The first is hemostasis during cardiac surgical procedures[6] and operations for splenic trauma. In these settings the hemostatic capacity of fibrin sealant is used to control bleeding tissues. The second approved indication is the use of this agent as a tissue sealant. It is approved to help facilitate closure and sealing of the colon at the time of colostomy closure. In this setting it can potentially reduce the rate of anastomotic leakage.

Fibrin sealant is stored in a refrigerator at 2° to 6° C. The commercial distributors (Tisseel VH, Baxter Corporation, Deerfield, Ill. and Hemaseel APR, Haemacure Corporation, Sarasota, Fla.) provide a special warmer and mixing device that can be used to facilitate rapid thawing and reconstitution of the powdered concentrates with diluent provided in the commercial kits. Preparation time is usually less than 20 minutes. There are multiple ways of applying this agent including (1) a dual-syringe device capable of providing fibrin sealant through a needle-tipped applicator to specific suture lines and (2) a gas-driven spray device (Fig. 3-1) that can apply small droplets of highly mixed material across broad surface areas. On mixing, the fibrinogen and thrombin form fibrin sealant within 30 seconds to 3 minutes. The initial liquid polymerizes rapidly to a firm material (Fig. 3-2). Newer applicators are also available including those capable of providing fibrin sealant endoscopically or through a minimally invasive surgical scope. The cost of the agent as presently distributed is approximately \$75 to \$100 for a 1 ml kit that is capable of producing 2 ml of the final fibrin sealant adhesive.

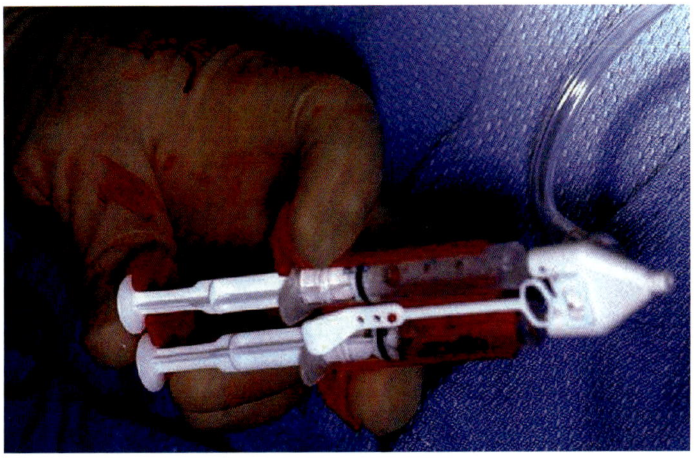

Figure 3-1 The gas-driven spray device for applying fibrin sealant as an aerosolized mist capable of covering large surface areas.

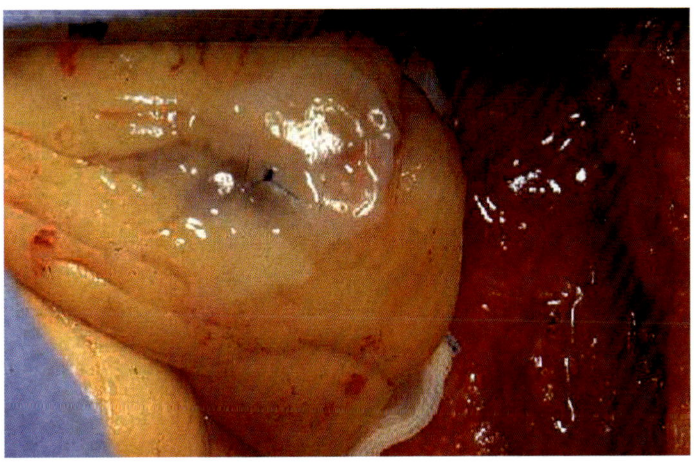

Figure 3-2 Fibrin sealant applied to the apex of the left ventricle to seal the myocardium after resection of an aneurysm.

Another commercial product employs the patient's own plasma as a source of fibrinogen to produce fibrin sealant that has been augmented by the addition of collagen. This product (CoStasis, Cohesion Technologies, Inc., Palo Alto, Calif.) has received FDA approval for use as an adjunct to hemostasis in a wide variety of surgical procedures including general, hepatic, and cardiovascular surgical procedures.[7,8] To prepare this agent, the patient's blood is obtained and a small tabletop centrifuge provided by the manufacturer is used to separate the patient's plasma and red cells. The plasma containing not only the patient's own fibrinogen but also platelets can then be combined with the bovine thrombin and collagen contained in a second syringe provided by the manufacturer. A dual-syringe applicator is used to apply the hemostatic agent. Although the concentrations of fibrinogen in this autologous system are less than those from manufactured commercial fibrin sealant, the material is augmented by the addition of collagen. The safety profile includes reduction of the risk of bloodborne disease transmission because autologous plasma is used but does involve the risks of using bovine thrombin. In rare instances, bovine thrombin has been reported to result in clotting abnormalities that can contribute significant coagulopathy.[9,10] In this setting the human body may form antibodies to thrombin, factor V, and other impurities in the bovine product that can cross-react with the patient's own clotting proteins. This reaction may cause a functional inactivation of the body's own clotting proteins and clotting pathways. Newer forms of bovine thrombin attempt to remove as many impurities as possible to minimize this problem.

Alternative modalities to the commercially provided forms of fibrin sealant include hospital-produced forms of fibrinogen that can be combined with bovine thrombin to produce fibrin sealant. The concentrated fibrinogen is prepared in the blood bank using cryoprecipitation[11] or in clinical laboratories using other chemical techniques.[12] These modalities produce fibrinogen concentrations between 15 and 35 mg/ml, which generally are lower than those available in commercial products. This can produce a fibrin sealant product that has less tensile and adhesive strength than commercial products. This product requires combination with thrombin to create fibrinogen. Thus it is dependent on the use of topical bovine thrombin, as no human thrombin stand-alone commercial product is presently available in the United States. The risk of antibody formation as a result of bovine thrombin also exists in this setting as a potential source of coagulopathy, particularly on reexposure to this type of product.[9,10] Another alternative can be found in the use of platelet gels (Medtronic, Minneapolis, Minn.). This technology involves the use of patient's plasma that is obtained during surgical procedures and can be concentrated using a centrifuge to create a plasma product that is rich in white blood cells and platelets. When combined with topical bovine thrombin, this platelet gel, rich in growth factors, can be used as a blood-clotting and wound-healing agent.[13,14]

Cyanoacrylate

Three commercial forms of cyanoacrylate are presently available. Two are available for skin closure, and one has been approved for embolization of arteriovenous malformations when presurgical devascularization is appropriate.

Presently the skin closure systems include 2-octyl cyanoacrylate (Dermabond, Ethicon, Somerville, N.J.) and n-butyl-2-cyanoacrylate (Indermil, United States Surgical, Norwalk, Conn.). These tissue adhesives are capable of bonding skin edges together, as cyanoacrylate in the presence of hydroxyl ions polymerizes in an exothermic reaction. The patients can sense this moderate release of heat as the material forms and creates a strong skin closure system. The materials are not absorbable and are sloughed from the surface of the skin as the upper dermal layers exfoliate 7 to 10 days after adhesive application. These materials are approved for external application only and are not to be used as internal tissue adhesives. Long-term internal use of cyanoacrylates may be associated with foreign body reactions, or carcinogenicity.[15] These cyanoacrylates are extremely strong adhesives that have been approved for closure of traumatic lacerations as well as easily approximated skin edges of surgical incisions. Such wounds could include emergency room lacerations and minimally invasive surgical incisions. The materials are not to be used in areas of high tension, mucosal membranes, or dense, natural hair. Because the agent functions by adhering to the superficial layers of the skin, application to high-tension areas could result in wound dehiscence. Although the glue is strong and creates a powerful bond to the superficial layers of the skin, the superficial layers of the skin itself may separate from deeper layers and can allow for wound dehiscence under high surface tension.

Both available commercial products for skin closure can be stored at room temperature. 2-Octyl cyanoacrylate comes as a single-dose crushable ampule, which is applied directly to the skin with direct contact of the applicator tip. The liquid polymerizes in a period of minutes on the skin surface. The company recommends three applications separated by 30 seconds each using a 1 cm band of application to each side of the skin incision. This material costs approximately $23 for a 0.5 ml ampule. N-butyl-2-cyanoacrylate is supplied in a 0.5 g plastic ampule. The material can be dripped onto the skin edges (Fig. 3-3) without direct applicator skin contact, achieving significant strength in approximately 30 seconds. Although this particular material remains stable at room temperature for a period of up to 4 weeks, long-term storage should be provided in a refrigerator between 2° and 5° C. For both agents, wounds should be prepared as they would with any other form of skin closure. The wound should be carefully cleaned, and hemostasis should be achieved before application of the tissue adhesive. Appropriate skin approximation is essential prior to

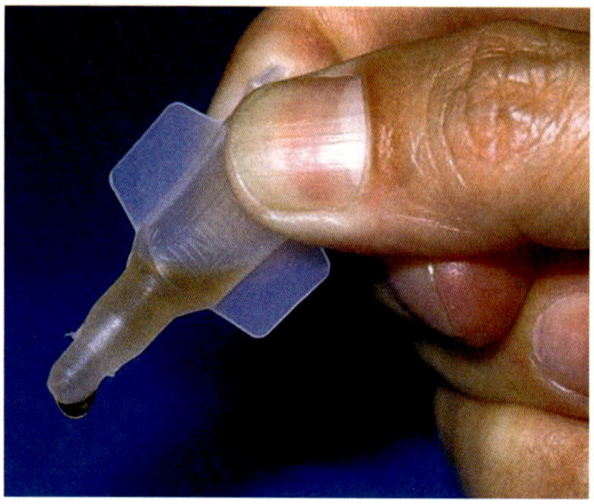

Figure 3-3 The applicator presently available for applying n-butyl-2-cyanoacrylate to skin incisions.

application of the cyanoacrylate; to achieve this, deep dermal sutures to enhance cosmesis and secure closure are recommended. Closure of the skin using these agents may be less painful and less emotionally traumatic, particularly in pediatric patients.[16-18] Cosmetic appearance is equivalent to that of wounds closed with sutures alone. Thus cyanoacrylates may be a valuable method of skin closure in cosmetic facial and plastic reconstructive surgery.[19]

The third available cyanoacrylate, n-butyl-2-cyanoacrylate, which recently received FDA approval for treatment of arteriovenous malformations, is also available for angiographic use (Trufill, Cordis Neurovascular, Inc., Miami Lakes, Fla.). This form of cyanoacrylate is provided in a system with tantalum powder so that the adhesive is radiopaque and can be placed with a super selective catheter delivery system under fluoroscopic guidance.[20] The material is indicated for the embolization of cerebral arteriovenous malformations when presurgical devascularization is desired. The long-term safety and effectiveness of this material have not been established, and that is why it is presently approved for temporary presurgical devascularization alone. The agent is so strong that caution needs to be taken to avoid gluing of the catheter delivery system to the arteriovenous malformation.

Bovine Collagen and Thrombin

The combination of bovine collagen and thrombin is provided as a hemostatic device that when used at the site of active bleeding is capable of achieving hemostasis. The bovine collagen and thrombin combination causes fibrinogen at the bleeding site to become fibrin and produces a clot. The collagen matrix swells by approximately 20% within a period of 10 minutes, adding to the tamponade effect of the hemostatic device. The risks of using bovine thrombin are in this product, specifically a coagulopathy that may occur as the human body manufactures antibodies against bovine thrombin or factor V. These antibodies may cross-react with human clotting proteins, producing a deficiency that may

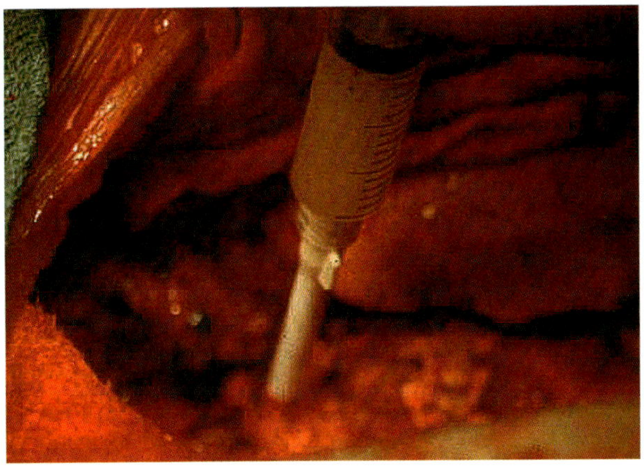

Figure 3-4 Application of bovine thrombin and collagen to the site of bleeding in repeat cardiac surgery.

cause a clinical coagulopathy.[9,10] This may be particularly important upon second exposure and should be considered by clinicians prior to re-exposure. The system is biodegradable and absorbed by the body within approximately 6 to 8 weeks.

The material is approved as a hemostatic device for active bleeding and is particularly effective in cardiovascular[21] and spinal procedures but is also approved as an adjunct to achieve hemostasis at all areas of surgical bleeding.[22] It is not recommended for ophthalmologic procedures because of the 20% expansion of the gelatin matrix.

The material is stored at room temperature, and reconstitution involves mixing the bovine thrombin with the collagen matrix. This takes approximately 5 minutes of preparation time. The single-syringe applicator system is then ready and is capable of delivering the toothpaste-like material to sites of active bleeding (Fig. 3-4). Pressure can be applied to the material with a moist sponge, which will not stick to the agent, as the material itself sticks only to sites of active bleeding where fibrinogen is present. The manufacturer (FloSeal, Baxter Corporation, Deerfield, Ill.) suggests that a polymerization time of 3 minutes be allowed to achieve maximum hemostasis with this material. Repeat applications to a site that has not been completely controlled can be performed by inserting the applicator tip so that it penetrates the previously applied material and delivers additional new product directly at the site of bleeding. The cost of this agent is $120 for a 3 ml kit.

Polyethylene Glycol Polymers

There are two polyethylene glycol (PEG) polymer systems now available for surgical use: (1) a light-activated system for pneumostasis at the time of lung resection and (2) a two-component PEG polymer system available for sealing blood vessels at the time of vascular anastomosis.

The light-activated PEG polymer was approved as a pneumostatic device and can be used to provide lung sealing at the time of lung resection.[23,24] The long-term effects of this agent are not known, and a slight (not statistically significant) increase in infection rate was noted in patients on whom this sealant was used.

The light-activated agent is stored at −20° to −4° C and is applied in a three-step process. The lung is prepared with a primer liquid that is rubbed into the pulmonary parenchyma with a wand applicator. This is followed by the application of the PEG polymer itself and light activation using a light source and cable. The application time is approximately 10 to 15 minutes. Studies in animals indicate that approximately one third of this material is still present in rats approximately 6 months after implantation. The cost of the agent is $450 for an 8 ml kit. The material is designed for thoracic surgery and is particularly useful with delicate pulmonary tissues (FocalSeal-L, Genzyme Biosurgery, Cambridge, Mass.).

The second PEG polymer system is a two-component polymer that is approved for sealing blood vessels and is useful for needle holes at the time of anastomoses between blood vessels or vascular grafts.[25] The material is a synthetic hydrogel that is formed using a two-component applicator capable of applying the two PEG polymers to the site of vascular anastomosis. As with other vascular sealants, it is important not to inject these materials directly into a blood vessel, as they can have an embolic effect. This material is presently distributed (CoSeal, Cohesion Technologies, Inc., Palo Alto, Calif.) as an adjunct to vascular hemostasis at the time of these surgical procedures. The material is stored at 2° to 8° C and is provided in a kit containing the two PEG polymers as well as the applicator system. The material is sprayed on the anastomoses from a distance of approximately 3 cm (Fig. 3-5), and polymerization requires approximately 60 seconds. The material is absorbed in the body in less than 4 weeks. The material is provided in 2, 4, and 8 ml kits. A mild skin sensitization reaction has been noted in animal models.

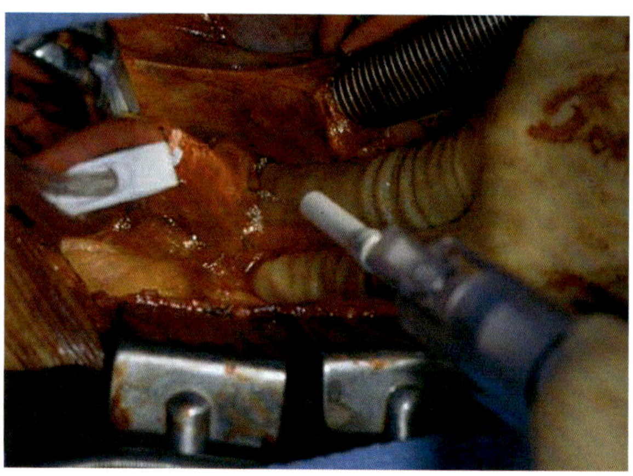

Figure 3-5 Simultaneous application of two PEG polymers to an aortic valve aortotomy closure suture line prior to pressurization of the aorta during cardiac valve replacement surgery.

Albumin Cross-Linked With Glutaraldehyde

This two-component surgical adhesive is composed of purified bovine serum albumin and glutaraldehyde. The glutaraldehyde molecules are capable of covalently bonding the bovine serum albumin molecules to themselves as well as to tissue proteins at the site of vascular anastomoses. The material is biodegradable over a period of months. This adhesive should not be used in patients with a history of allergy to bovine products. Because the agent is often used near open blood vessels and changes from a liquid to a solid form quite rapidly, great care should be used not to allow the material to occlude branch blood vessels or form embolic clots. The agent is often applied around circumferential anastomoses and thus, similar to a running suture, would not permit anastomotic growth. Therefore it should not be used in a pediatric population with continued growth potential. The glutaraldehyde in the material is capable of causing nerve injury, and therefore caution should be taken to avoid application to nerve tissues or in proximity to nerve structures such as the sinuatrial node of the heart. Long-term follow-up with respect to the effects of this material is pending.

Albumin cross-linked with glutaraldehyde is a strong, rapidly forming adhesive that has been approved for sealing large vascular anastomoses (Fig. 3-6).[26,27] It can also be used to glue layers of aorta back together and to strengthen tissues at the time of repair of aortic dissections. This material should be used sparingly, as excess application can result in tissue distortion as well as potential necrosis or redissection.[28,29]

The agent can be stored for long periods at temperatures of 25° C or less but should not be frozen. The two-component system is provided in an applicator gun that allows mixing of the glutaraldehyde and bovine serum albumin components. The material begins to polymerize as it reaches the tip of the applicator gun. An additional applicator extension is provided to assist in getting the materials to more confined spaces. Assembly of the gun and component takes

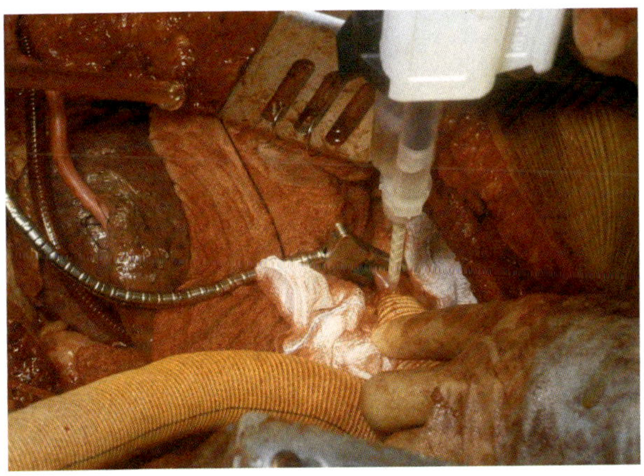

Figure 3-6 Application of albumin cross-linked with glutaraldehyde to an anastomosis between a Dacron synthetic graft and the aorta at the time of thoracic aortic aneurysm resection.

a few minutes, and the material is capable of polymerizing within 30 seconds to 2 minutes. The manufacturer (BioGlue, CryoLife, Inc., Kennesaw, Ga.) provides the material at a cost of approximately $450 for a 5 ml kit.

Clinical Algorithms

Hemostasis

These clinical algorithms for the use of tissue adhesives are based on our personal experience over a number of years using these agents. These sections will deal with both on-label and off-label uses of tissue adhesives. The clinician should be aware that the approved FDA indications for each of these agents were reviewed in previous discussions.

Control of bleeding in the operating room depends on the characteristics of the bleeding diathesis itself. Specifically, is the bleeding arterial or venous and is it diffuse or localized? Also the extent of the bleeding is an important factor. Clearly none of the available tissue adhesives are likely to be effective in a setting with massive bleeding where sutures or even patches may be required. Even some major forms of bleeding, however, can be dealt with using tissue adhesives. Fig. 3-7 suggests that fibrin sealant and bovine collagen and thrombin are agents that significantly improve the ability to control surgical bleeding. Fibrin sealant is capable of controlling diffuse bleeding, particularly that which would be encountered at the time of reoperative surgery for adhesions. The material can be sprayed over diffuse surface areas in a well-mixed, thinly applied, and efficiently delivered layer. This method is particularly effective if supported by tissue-to-tissue contact between layers after spraying the material. Specific localized applications of fibrin sealant can be performed by a dual-syringe, needle-tipped applicator, but strong bleeding will wash the liquid fibrin

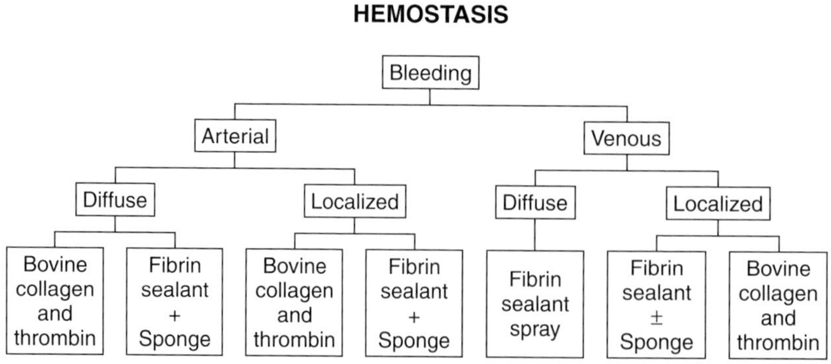

Figure 3-7 Algorithm for use of tissue adhesives to achieve hemostasis.

sealant away before its polymerization. Thus significant localized arterial or venous bleeding may not be controlled by the fibrin sealant. In this setting, fibrin sealant is best delivered with a carrier sponge.[30] Available products include gelatin or collagen sheets that can be coated with fibrin sealant on one side to deliver the fibrin sealant to the site of active bleeding while pressure is applied to the sponge. This is an effective means of controlling hemorrhage. It will be successful if the bleeding can be stopped with pressure for several minutes while the fibrin sealant polymerizes. Fibrin sealant can also be used prophylactically to seal vascular anastomoses and prevent bleeding.[31] In other words, after a vascular anastomosis is completed, but prior to pressurization, the anastomosis can be coated with fibrin sealant. After this material has polymerized, the anastomosis can be repressurized with a minimal amount of bleeding. This is particularly effective for delicate tissues or for polytetrafluoroethylene grafts that have been sewn in place with polypropylene sutures and that could bleed from needle holes. Use of fibrin sealant in this setting is almost 100% effective in preventing bleeding and reducing the time required for hemostasis after the synthetic graft is pressurized.

Collagen-thrombin is a powerful hemostatic agent that is particularly effective because of its ability to be combined with manual pressure. This is provided through a moist operating room pad or sponge, a traditional technique frequently used by surgeons to achieve hemostasis. Because this product is a solid material and not liquid, it can be applied to a site with relatively active bleeding and not be washed away by the source of blood flow. Pressure with a moist sponge can be immediately applied after the thick, toothpaste-like material has been applied to keep it in place and to facilitate hemostasis. In this setting major venous bleeding can be controlled, and in some settings even significant arterial hemorrhage can be treated successfully. This agent is more effective at dealing with localized bleeding than with bleeding that occurs over a major surface area. This agent requires active bleeding to provide a source of fibrinogen, which will combine with collagen and thrombin to form a collagen and fibrin plug. Thus it is not effective for prophylactic use. In other words, it cannot be applied to a depressurized vascular anastomosis when there is no active bleeding, as it will not be activated. The required blood source in this setting is missing, and no fibrinogen is available for activation by the commercial product.

Vascular Sealing

This section is intended to help with the sealing of vascular anastomoses that involve native blood vessels or vascular grafts. Fig. 3-8 addresses two situations: (1) choosing the appropriate agent before the vessel has been pressurized and has developed active bleeding and (2) choosing the appropriate agent after the vessel has been pressurized and active bleeding may be present.

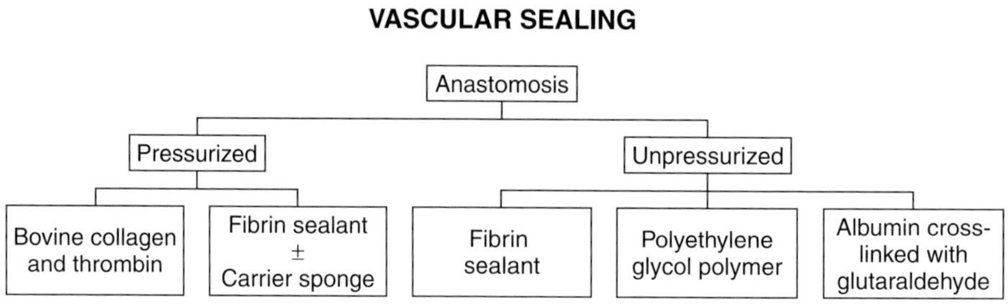

Figure 3-8 Algorithm for the proper application of tissue adhesives to vascular anastomoses.

There are three good choices available at present for sealing blood vessels that are not pressurized and that as yet have not developed active bleeding. Fibrin sealant can be applied in this setting using either the needle-tipped applicator or gas-driven spray applicator to coat the anastomosis and seal the anastomotic tissue line as well as needle holes.[31] Fibrin sealant is a relatively weak adhesive, so it will not hold the anastomosis together. The anastomosis needs to have been adequately sewn with good technical skills. However, the sealant is capable of reinforcing weaker tissues to prevent bleeding and sealing needle holes such as those seen in polytetrafluoroethylene vascular grafts when polypropylene sutures are used. Approximately 2 to 3 minutes should be allowed for the fibrin sealant to set before repressurizing the anastomosis so that maximum effectiveness is achieved from the fibrin sealant. In this situation the sealant not only achieves a sealing effect but also brings its inherent hemostatic capacity to bear.

Another reasonable choice for sealing vascular anastomoses is the dual PEG polymer system that can be applied through a spray tip applicator. This system allows a clear layer of hydrogel to coat the anastomosis. In the unpressurized anastomotic setting with no active bleeding, at least 60 seconds of polymerization time is recommended for this synthetic sealant to fully function. This agent is capable of sealing needle holes.[25] It does not have any inherent clotting ability. Thus, if bleeding develops after the anastomosis is repressurized, other modalities should be used to supplement this technique to achieve final hemostasis. This material provides a jellylike coating but does not provide strong anastomotic bonding.

Finally, an unpressurized anastomosis can be sealed using albumin cross-linked with glutaraldehyde.[26,27] This agent has a strong strength profile. Small amounts can be used sparingly with the gun applicator to achieve vascular sealing. The additional extension on the applicator tip will allow a less liquid material with more viscosity to be applied to the anastomosis in a more controlled fashion. The agent should be used sparingly and should perhaps not be used at the site of polytetrafluoroethylene anastomosis because there is a risk that the material could penetrate needle holes and function as a vascular embolic nidus. This material adds significant strength and reinforcement to an anastomosis. It will not permit tissue growth and should be avoided in growing pediatric patients. No clear evidence of significant tissue necrosis as a result of using this agent presently exists. Concerns about potential false aneurysm formation and recurrent vascular dissections using this agent are described in the literature.[28,29]

Both the PEG polymer and the albumin cross-linked with glutaraldehyde are relatively ineffective in settings that are moist. They require dry environments to polymerize appropriately with anastomotic tissues and cannot be used successfully at a site of active bleeding.

When one is dealing with a pressurized anastomosis that is actively bleeding, a setting similar to that described for hemostasis (see Fig. 3-7) occurs. Fibrin sealant delivered with a carrier sponge to the specific site of active bleeding and kept in place for a period of minutes may be useful.[30] This is opposed to liquid fibrin sealant, which may be washed away with a stream of blood. Similarly, bovine collagen and thrombin can be delivered to the anastomotic site as a solid matrix that combined with pressure from a moist sponge can tamponade the bleeding and achieve hemostasis after pressure has been applied for 2 to 3 minutes.[21,22]

Thus the major decision in this algorithm is the presence of an unpressurized dry anastomosis versus a pressurized actively bleeding, moist anastomotic environment. The agents should be chosen with respect to this dichotomy as well as with respect to the strength and safety profiles of the agents themselves.

Tissue Apposition

The algorithm for tissue approximation is provided in Fig. 3-9. Two different cyanoacrylate preparations are now available for closure of superficial skin lacerations or incisions and for reinforcement of deeper incisions that have first been closed with deep dermal sutures. The available choices are 2-octyl cyanoacrylate and n-butyl-2-cyanoacrylate. These agents are effective at closing skin

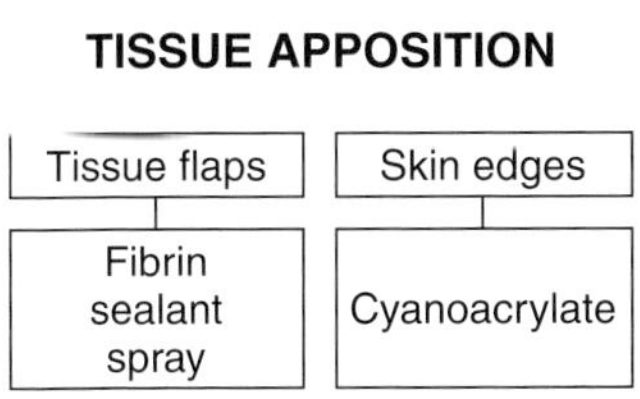

Figure 3-9 Algorithm for the proper application of tissue adhesives to achieve skin flap or graft apposition.

defects in low-tension areas. They are particularly useful for traumatic lacerations treated in the emergency room[16-18] or in cosmetic surgery in the hands of a skilled surgeon capable of approximating subdermal and deep dermal layers with sutures prior to skin closure with cyanoacrylate.[19] The 2-octyl cyanoacrylate is applied directly to the skin from a crushable ampule. Multiple layers of this product are applied separated by 30 second polymerization intervals. The n-butyl-2-cyanoacrylate is applied through a dropper that does not require skin contact. These agents both polymerize over a period of approximately 30 seconds. Wounds closed with these agents should be prepared as with any surgical skin closure. Specifically the wound should be thoroughly cleaned and the skin edges freshened. All areas of bleeding should be controlled before skin closure. These agents will be effective only in areas that are not subjected to major skin tension. These materials can only approximate the wounds for 7 to 10 days. After this time the superficial layers of skin to which the adhesive is adherent are sloughed. The cyanoacrylates are not presently available for internally gluing tissue flaps together, because of safety concerns.[15]

The only agent presently available for the apposition of tissues such as flaps and skin grafts is fibrin sealant. The safety profile of this agent in internal use is relatively good. It can be used to effect tissue adherence and to eliminate potential seroma spaces. It is also an effective hemostatic and lymphostatic agent for prevention of leakage from capillaries and lymphatic vessels.[30] In this setting skill is required to use the fibrin sealant properly. Surgical areas must be prepared so that after the fibrin sealant is sprayed, the tissues to be in contact are immediately approximated and then not disturbed.[32] In this way, excellent tissue apposition will occur, and the potential space will be sealed.[33] If, however, a delay occurs between spraying the fibrin sealant on the intended surfaces such that tissue contact between the two surfaces to be apposed does not occur immediately and polymerization of the glue occurs prior to contact, then the sealant actually functions as an antiadhesive. The tissues will not stick together, and a significant potential for seroma formation will exist. Thus paradoxically the use of fibrin sealant in this setting when tissue apposition is delayed can actually create a worse potential for seroma formation than would have been there had the sealant not been used at all. Even if the tissues are rapidly apposed so polymerization occurs while the tissues are in contact, disrupting the tissue bond by pulling one tissue away from the other can again cause the antiadhesive effect. For example, picking up the superficial skin layer with a forceps to apply additional sutures can cause disruption of this bond and create an antiadhesive effect of the fibrin sealant that could also potentiate seroma formation.

The best way of applying fibrin sealant to achieve the maximum apposition effect is to preplace a latticework of subcutaneous or cutaneous monofilament sutures that can be pulled tight immediately after placement of the sealant.[32] This is quickly followed by pressure on the flap to cause apposition of the flap and underlying tissues. This allows for polymerization of the two layers immediately while the tissues are in contact and avoids tissue disruption by eliminating the need for later placement of sutures.

Fibrin sealant can also be used to aid with the fixation and placement of split-thickness skin grafts.[30] It is an extremely effective way of placing grafts in areas that might not normally provide adequate nutrient support for graft survival. Unusual areas on the head and neck can thus be used to support skin grafts without large bolus dressings or the need of suture fixation. The fibrin sealant is capable of fixing the skin graft without large bolus dressings. It is important in this setting to avoid excessive use of fibrin sealant, as too thick a layer of the material in between the underlying tissues and the thin skin graft will block nutrient flow from the underlying bed to the skin graft itself. This may significantly reduce graft survival.

Pneumostasis

The leakage of air from the parenchyma of the lung or from the tracheobronchial tree can be a significant challenge for the surgeon. Placement of additional sutures in this fragile environment may not be rewarded by any significant improvement. Therefore any mechanism that can stop air leaks from staple lines or sutured closures may be of significant value.

In the pulmonary parenchyma itself (Fig. 3-10), there are two potentially useful agents. First, light-activated PEG polymer can be used to seal fragile staple lines and is particularly useful with delicate emphysematous tissues as might be encountered in lung volume reduction surgery.[23,24] This modality requires placement of a primer prior to addition of the light-activated PEG polymer and may require several minutes for application. A significant improvement in control of immediate air leaks as well as of postoperative chest tube air leaks has been noted using this agent. Thus it appears to be useful in achieving more effective pneumostasis from the parenchyma of the lung.

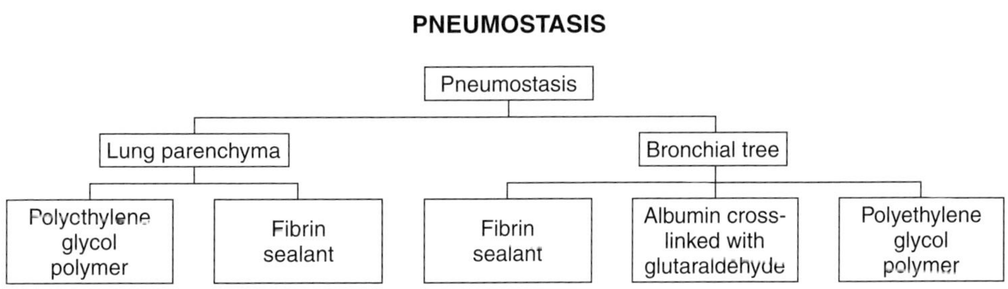

Figure 3-10 Algorithm for the proper application of tissue adhesives to achieve pneumostasis of the lung parenchyma or tracheobronchial tree.

There are reports of using fibrin sealant in a similar setting.[1] Fibrin sealant, however, is a relatively weak adhering adhesive. Large changes in the surface contour of the lung may occur between lung deflation at the time of sealant application and significant lung reinflation after sealing. Significant stress during reinflation and lung expansion may disrupt fibrin sealant bonds to the surface of the lung. Recent reports suggest that spray application of fibrin sealant across a larger area of the pulmonary parenchyma may be more effective in this setting. This technique may reduce the problem of changing lung contour and improve the effectiveness of this agent.

The two agents just discussed may be useful in closure of the bronchial tree, and anecdotal reports from Europe have suggested that albumin cross-linked with glutaraldehyde also may be used in this setting. It may be important to establish that the use of this agent in this setting is not associated with any significant tissue necrosis or fibrosis.

Lymphostasis

In a variety of settings involving dissection of lymphatics for tumor resections, lymphatic leak may be a significant contributor to postoperative morbidity, including seroma formation, infection, and wound dehiscence. An agent capable of providing lymphostasis (Fig. 3-11) and of eliminating potential spaces by causing skin to adhere to underlying tissue may be of significant value. Fibrin sealant when properly used is an effective lymphatic sealant and can be used to effect tissue adherence and eliminate potential spaces.[30,32,33] It is important to prepare the tissues so that skin closure is achieved immediately after the sealant is sprayed. In this setting a latticework of sutures is pulled tight immediately after the sealant is sprayed to approximate the skin edges, and pressure is applied to the skin to cause it to be approximated to the underlying tissue and tissue adhesive.[32] Great care should be taken to avoid any pulling of the skin away from the underlying tissues because disruption at this point, after sealant polymerization, will have a significant antiadhesive effect. This capability may be extremely important in radical lymphatic surgical dissections for malignancies in the head, neck, axilla, and groin.

Vascular Embolization

The FDA recently has approved n-butyl-2-cyanoacrylate as a means of decreasing blood flow to arteriovenous malformations prior to surgical resection (Fig. 3-12). This agent requires skilled application using angiographic techniques dependent on fluoroscopy.[20] In addition, the approval for this application is dependent on the assumption that these malformations will be resected at a later date by a neurosurgeon. Thus concerns about the long-term effects of the cyanoacrylate are not warranted because the agent itself is removed surgically from the patient soon after its use.

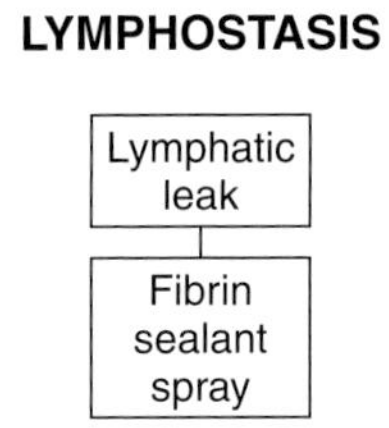

Figure 3-11 Algorithm for the proper application of tissue adhesives to achieve lymphostasis and eliminate the possibility of seroma formation.

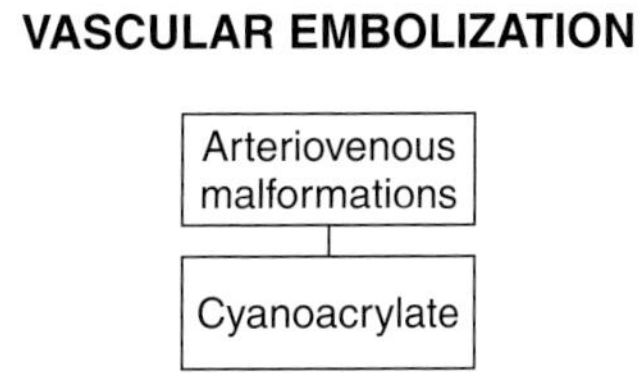

Figure 3-12 Algorithm for the proper application of tissue adhesives to achieve vascular embolization of arteriovenous malformations.

Conclusion

Present

In this chapter the appropriate on-label indications for the five new families of tissue adhesives have been described. These agents are particularly valuable in view of the greater technical challenges presented by minimally invasive surgery. Individual agents have been reviewed in depth. Algorithms for the use of these materials to achieve hemostasis, vascular sealing, tissue apposition, pneumostasis, lymphostasis, and vascular embolization have been provided (see Figs. 3-7 to 3-12). These algorithms combine on-label and off-label indications for these agents.

Appropriate use of these materials in cosmetic surgery should reduce tissue trauma, swelling, and ecchymosis in the early postoperative period as well as improve healing and effect more cosmetically attractive outcomes. Subsequent chapters in this book will deal in-depth with the use of agents in specific procedures.

Future

Future developments in the field of tissue adhesives will be centered in at least two areas. First, safer and more effective agents are in the early stages of development or clinical testing. These materials will be second-generation agents similar to those presently available or will be third-generation materials with significantly enhanced tissue adhesive capabilities. Second, tissue adhesive may be used in a capacity other than as a pure single-purpose surgical glue. Fibrin sealant, for example, has significant drug delivery capabilities that may allow it to be used to deliver antibiotics, growth factors, chemotherapeutic agents, or local anesthetics.[34] Thus tissue adhesives may be used not only for gluing but also for delivering drugs. These agents may have important roles in tissue engineering and cellular growth as well.

ACKNOWLEDGMENT

We would like to thank Kristen Faircloth and Sylvie Martinez for their assistance in the preparation of the manuscript.

REFERENCES

1. Spotnitz WD, Falstrom JK, Rodeheaver GT. The role of sutures and fibrin sealant in wound healing. Surg Clin North Am 77:651-669, 1997.
2. Spotnitz WD. History of tissue adhesives. In Sierra D, Saltz R, eds. Surgical Adhesives and Sealants, Current Technology and Applications. Lancaster, Pa: Technomic Publishing, 1996.
3. Spotnitz WD, Burks S, Mercer D. Clinical indications for surgical tissue adhesives. In Lewandrowski K-U, Wise DL, Trantolo DH, Gresser JD, Yaszemski MJ, Altobelli DE, eds. Tissue Engineering and Biodegradable Equivalents: Scientific and Clinical Applications. New York: Marcel Dekker, 2002.
4. Spotnitz W, Mercer D, Burks S. Tissue adhesives and hemostats: New tools for the surgeon. In Chaudry M, Pocius AV, eds. Adhesion Science and Engineering—2: Surfaces, Chemistry and Applications. Amsterdam: Elsevier Science, 2002.
5. Spotnitz WD, Burks S. Use of tissue sealants in cardiac surgery. In Franco KL, Verrier ED, eds. Advanced Therapy in Cardiac Surgery, 2nd ed. Hamilton, Ontario, BC: Marcel Dekker, 2003.
6. Rousou J, Gonzalez-Lavin L, Cosgrove D, Weldon C, Hess P, Joyce L, Bergsland J, Gazzaniga A. Randomized clinical trial of fibrin sealant in patients undergoing resternotomy or reoperation after cardiac operations. J Thorac Cardiovasc Surg 97:194-203, 1989.
7. Chapman W, Sherman R, Boyce S, Malawer M, Hill A, Buncke G, Block J, Fung J, Clavien P, Lee K, Lebovic G, Wren S, Diethrich E, Goldstein R. A novel collagen-based composite offers effective hemostasis for multiple surgical indications: Results of a randomized controlled trial. Surgery 129:445-450, 2001.
8. Chapman W, Clavien P, Fung J, Khanna A, Bonham A. Effective control of hepatic bleeding using a novel collagen-based composite combined with autologous plasma: Results of a randomized controlled trial. Arch Surg 13:1200-1204, 2000.
9. Nichols WL, Daniels TM, Fisher PK, Antibodies to bovine thrombin and coagulation factor V associated with the use of topical bovine thrombin or fibrin glue: A frequent finding. Blood 82:59a, 1993.
10. Ortel TL, Mercer MC, Thames EH, Moore, KD, Lawson JH. Immunologic impact and clinical outcomes after surgical exposure to bovine thrombin. Ann Surg 233:88-96, 2001.
11. Spotnitz WD, Mintz PD, Avery N, Bithell TC, Kaul S, Nolan SP. Fibrin glue from stored human plasma: An inexpensive and efficient method for local blood bank preparation. Am Surg 53:460-464, 1987.
12. Siedentop K, Harris D, Ham K, Sanchez B. Extended experimental and preliminary surgical findings with autologous fibrin tissue adhesive made from patient's own blood. Laryngoscope 96:1062-1064, 1986.
13. Hill AG, Hood AG, Reeder GD, Potter PS, Iverson LIG, Keating RF, Speir AM, Lefrak EA. Perioperative autologous sequestration II: A differential centrifugation technique for autologous component therapy: Methods and results. Am Acad Cardiovasc Perfus 14:122-125, 1993.
14. Hood, AG, Hill AG, Reeder GD, Potter PS, Iverson LIG, Keating RF, Speir AM, Lefrak EA. Perioperative autologous sequestration III: A new physiologic glue with wound healing properties. Am Acad Cardiovasc Perfus 14:126-129, 1993.
15. Samson D, Marshall D. Carcinogenic potential of isobutyl-2-cyanoacrylate. J Neurosurg 65:571-572, 1986.
16. Quinn J, Drzewiecki A, Li M, Stiell I, Sutcliffe T, Elmslie T, Wood W. A randomized, controlled trial comparing a tissue adhesive with suturing in the repair of pediatric facial lacerations. Ann Emerg Med 22:1130-1135, 1993.

17. Quinn J, Wells G, Sutcliffe T, Jarmuske M, Maw J, Stiel I, Johns P. A randomized trial comparing octyl-cyanoacrylate tissue adhesive and sutures in the management of lacerations. JAMA 277:1527-1530, 1997.
18. Schonauer, F, Pereira J, La Rusca I, Harris J, Cullen K. Use of Indermil tissue adhesive for closure of superficial skin lacerations in children. Minerva Chir 56:427-429, 2001.
19. Toriumi DM, O'Grady K, Devang D, Bagal A. Use of octyl-2-cyanoacrylate for skin closure in facial plastic surgery. Plast Reconstr Surg 102:2209-2219, 1998.
20. The n-BCA Trial Investigators. N-butyl cyanoacrylate embolization of cerebral arteriovenous malformations: Results of a prospective, randomized, multi-center trial. AJNR Am J Neuroradiol 23:748-755, 2002.
21. Oz MC, Cosgrove DM, Badduke BR, Hill JD, Flannery M, Palumbo R. Topic N, and The Fusion Matrix Study Group. Controlled clinical trial of a novel hemostatic agent in cardiac surgery. Ann Thorac Surg 69:1376-1382, 2000.
22. Reuthebuch O, Lachat ML, Vogt O, Schurr U, Turina M. FloSeal: A new hemostyptic agent in peripheral vascular surgery. Clin Cardiovasc Surg 29:204-206, 2000.
23. Ranger WR, Halpin D, Sawhney AS, Lyman M, Locicero J. Pneumostasis of experimental air leaks with a new photo polymerized synthetic tissue sealant. Am Surg 63:788-795, 1997.
24. Wain JC, Kaiser LR, Johnstone DW, Yang SC, Wright CD, Friedberg JS, Feins RH, Heitmiller RF, Mathisen DJ, Selwyn MR. Trial of a novel synthetic sealant in preventing air leaks after lung resection. Ann Thorac Surg 71:1623-1629, 2001.
25. Glickman M, Gheissari A, Money S, Martin J, Ballard JL. CoSeal Multicenter Vascular Surgery Study Group. A polymeric sealant inhibits anastomotic suture hole bleeding more rapidly than Gelfoam/thrombin: Results of a randomized controlled trial. Arch Surg 137:326-331, 2001.
26. Hewitt, CW, Marra SW, Kann BR, Tran HS, Puc MM, Chrizanowski FA Jr, Tran JL, Lenz SD, Cilley JH Jr, Simonetti VA, DelRossi AJ. BioGlue surgical adhesive for thoracic aortic repair during coagulopathy: Efficacy and histopathology. Ann Thorac Surg 71:1609-1612, 2001.
27. Raanani E, Latter DA, Errett LE, Bonneau DB, Leclerc Y, Salasidis GC. Use of "BioGlue" in aortic surgical repair. Ann Thorac Surg 72:638-640, 2001.
28. Bingley, JA, Gardner MAH, Stafford EG, Mau TK, Pohlner PG, Tam RKW, Jalali H, Tesar PJ, O'Brien MF. Late complications of tissue glues in aortic surgery. Ann Thorac Surg 69:1764-1768, 2000.
29. Kazui, T, Washiyama N, Bashar AHM, Terada H, Suzuki K, Yamashita K, Takinami M. Role of biologic glue repair of proximal aortic dissection in the development of early and midterm redissection of the aortic root. Ann Thorac Surg 72:509-514, 2001.
30. Spotnitz WD. Fibrin sealant in the United States: Clinical use at the University of Virginia. Thromb Haemost 74:482-485, 1995.
31. Schenk W, Goldthwaite Jr C, Burks S, Spotnitz W. Fibrin sealant facilitates hemostasis in arteriovenous polytetrafluoroethylene grafts for renal dialysis access. Am Surg 68:728-732, 2002.
32. Moore MM, Nguyen DHD, Spotnitz WD. Fibrin sealant reduces serous drainage and allows earlier drain removal after axillary dissection: A randomized prospective trial. Am Surg 63:97-102, 1997.
33. Moore M, Burak Jr W, Nelson E, Kearney T, Simmons R, Mayers L, Spotnitz W. Fibrin sealant reduces the duration and amount of fluid drainage following axillary dissection: A randomized prospective clinical trial. J Am Coll Surg 192:591-599, 2001.
34. MacPhee M, Singh M, Brady R, Akhyani N, Liau G, Lasa C, Hue C, Best A, Drohan W. Fibrin sealant: A versatile delivery vehicle for drugs and biologics. In Sierra D, Saltz R, eds. Surgical Adhesives and Sealants, Current Technology and Applications. Lancaster, Pa: Technomic Publishing, 1996.

CHAPTER

4

Autologous Platelet-Rich Plasma in Facial Aesthetic Surgery

Ross A. Clevens, M.D.

This chapter presents an overview of the use of platelet-rich plasma (PRP) in facial aesthetic surgery and reevaluates my experience with autologous preparations of PRP and platelet-poor plasma (fibrin glue) in over 500 facial plastic surgery cases. PRP is a gel that uses a high concentration of platelets and the inherent concentration of fibrinogen harvested by the centrifugal separation of autologous whole blood. This wound sealant has an array of cytokines and mediators that increase recollagenation, accelerate epidermal and epithelial regeneration, promote angiogenesis, enhance wound strength, hasten hemostasis, improve tissue regeneration, decrease dermal scarring, and facilitate remodeling. The objective of this chapter is to establish the role of PRP and fibrin glue in facial plastic and reconstructive surgery with particular reference to aesthetic facial surgery.

The Biology of Platelet-Rich Plasma and Wound Healing

Every surgical procedure creates controlled tissue injury. The body responds to this trauma by initiating the healing cascade by first forming a clot to repair the insult. This clot creates a hemostatic barrier or seal at the wound site to halt blood loss and prevent foreign organisms and materials from entering the wound. The clot also serves as a scaffold into which new repair cells migrate and subsequently divide to permit tissue regeneration to proceed. These steps in the healing cascade are initiated and modulated by signal proteins found in the clot. These proteins are transported to the site of injury by the circulating blood; the plasma, leukocytes, and platelets orchestrate the healing cascade and repair process. The clot is composed of strands of fibrin from the fibrinogen, which is from the plasma and the membranes of activated platelets.[1] It follows that increasing the concentration of these signal proteins at the injury site may enhance the healing rate; the application of PRP achieves such an increase in signal proteins and bioactive molecules at the wound.

PRP is a volume of autologous plasma that has a concentration of platelets greater than baseline. Whereas normal platelet concentrations generally range from 150,000/μl to 350,000/μl, PRP concentrate exceeds 1 million/μl. Data suggest that the platelet concentration must exceed 1 million/μl for PRP to be biologically active.

PRP is a gel containing a high concentration of platelets and a native concentration of fibrinogen harvested by the centrifugal separation of autologous whole blood.[2-4] This gel is an autologous platelet-based wound sealant that functions as a hemostatic agent. This wound sealant has an array of cytokines and mediators that have been demonstrated in vitro and in vivo to increase recollagenation, accelerate epidermal and epithelial regeneration, promote angiogenesis, enhance wound strength, hasten hemostasis, improve tissue regeneration, decrease dermal scarring, and facilitate wound remodeling.[5]

PRP markedly increases the proliferative activity within a surgical wound. PRP also promotes continued cell-differentiated activities including ground substance formation, wound matrix proliferation, and mineral deposition.[6] Cytokines and mediators within platelet gel facilitate osteoblast-like cell regulation and fibroblastlike cell amplification.

Growth factors represent signals that organize and coordinate cellular proliferation. Most growth factors are large peptides or glycoproteins released from macrophages, neutrophils, lymphocytes, platelets, and fibroblasts. Growth factors bind to target cells at a specific cell surface receptor. Once activated, growth factors induce cell migration, division, and proliferation and chemotactically attract other wound-healing factors for rapid and active wound repair.

Platelet activation and function are characterized by the actions of the platelet alpha granule and the platelet dense granule. Platelet alpha granules release beta proteins that initiate the wound-healing cascade. This cascade activates fibroblasts, endothelial cells, and macrophages, which promotes the rapid repair of wounds. Important proteins comprising the alpha granule include platelet-derived growth factor (PDGF), transforming growth factor beta (TGF-β), fibroblast growth factor (FGF), platelet-derived epidermal growth factor (PDEGF), platelet-derived angiogenesis factor (PDAF), platelet factor 4 (antiheparin factor, PF-4), platelet-activating factor (PAF), and insulin-like growth factor (IGF).

In addition, there are in excess of 200 named cytokine growth factors and mediators associated with the platelet. The topical application of the growth factors present in PRP enhances wound healing and optimizes the tensile strength of wounds. TGF-β has been demonstrated to increase collagen synthesis and decrease dermal scarring.

Platelet-dense granules carry vasoactive amines that increase microvascular permeability. This change in vascular permeability allows effector (activator or inhibitor) cells to enter the wound. This promotes phagocytic activity, while macrophages facilitate debridement and microbiologic surveillance. Important vasoactive amines associated with the platelet-dense granule include ionized calcium, adenosine diphosphate, histamine, epinephrine, and serotonin.

The clinical benefits of PRP include the release of concentrated wound-healing growth factors that enhance angiogenesis, increase collagenesis, improve wound strength, and hasten bone maturity. Fibrin deposition or augmented fibrin deposition enhances hemostasis and wound contracture. This has been associated with a reduction in postoperative pain, reduction in postoperative risk of infection, and improved wound healing.

Initially the procurement of PRP entailed the assistance of a perfusionist operating a cumbersome and costly cell-saver apparatus. Currently there are several proprietary ambulatory systems on the market that enable the rapid, reliable, and simple production of PRP at the time of outpatient aesthetic facial surgery including those from Harvest Technologies (Plymouth, Mass.) (Fig. 4-1), Secquire (Fig. 4-2) from Perfusion Partners and Associates, Inc. (PPAI, Fort Myers, Fla.), and 3I Implant Technologies (Fort Lauderdale, Fla.).

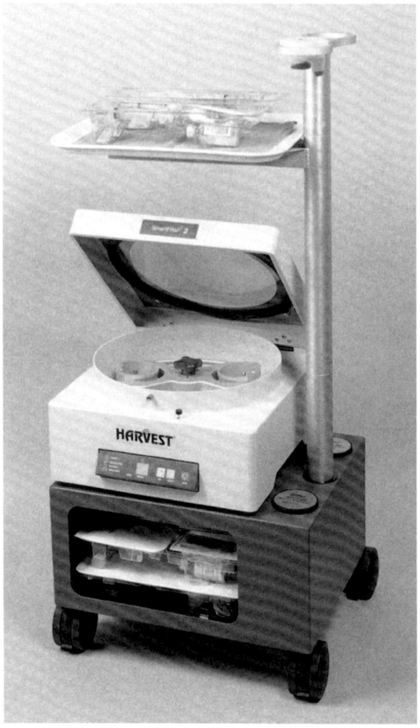

Figure 4-1 The Harvest ambulatory centrifugal system for the procurement of platelet-rich plasma.

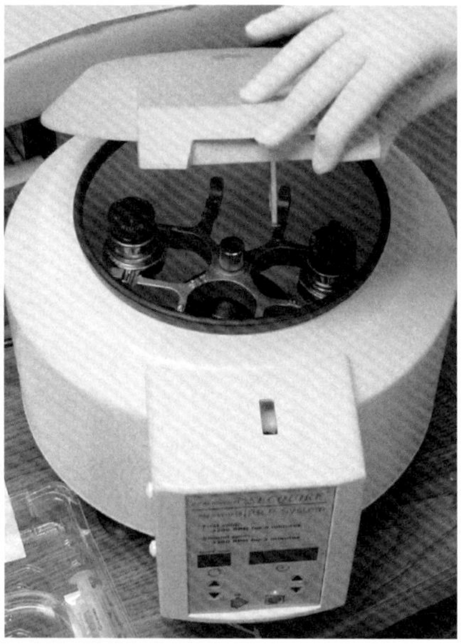

Figure 4-2 The Perfusion Partners mobile Secquire centrifuge for the production of platelet-rich plasma.

Because PRP is developed from autologous blood, it is inherently safe from transmissible diseases.[7] In contrast, as Man and Plosker[8] point out, the use of material derived from pooled blood products entails the risk of disease transmission in cosmetic surgery. There have been at least two case reports of disease transmission associated with the use of pooled fibrin glue, one involving parvovirus B19 infection[9] and another involving human immunodeficiency virus (HIV) infection.[10]

Indications for Use: A Review of the Clinical Literature

Some of the first clinical reports advocating PRP to modulate healing appear in the oral and maxillofacial surgery literature; it was used to enhance bone graft survival and to promote and accelerate osseointegration. PRP has been successful intraorally for site preparation, sinus lifts, and alveolar ridge augmentation. Soft tissue healing enhancement and rapid re-epithelialization have been documented by Marx et al.[11] Soft tissue dental applications further include palatal grafts, gingival flaps, and cosmetic dentistry soft tissue augmentations.

Monteleone et al.[12] reported enhanced healing of skin graft donor sites with PRP. Side-by-side skin grafts were harvested from patients creating defects in neighboring sites to assess the potential effect of PRP on acceleration of soft tissue healing and facilitation of wound re-epithelialization. PRP added topically to the de-epithelialized region significantly accelerated wound healing and decreased postoperative pain. The mechanism of enhanced healing was thought to be related to the release of PDGF and TGF-β as well as to a fibrin-rich base that facilitates early revascularization and a framework for epithelial migration.

Kerner[13] assessed postoperative healing in a series of patients undergoing functional endoscopic sinus surgery. Employing PRP as a form of postoperative packing, Kerner reported reduced time to remucosalization, less postoperative bleeding, and decreased postoperative patient discomfort. No PRP-related intranasal synechias were observed.

A review of the plastic surgery literature yields several recent important reports, most notably by Welsh,[14] Melmed,[15] Man et al.,[16] Oliver et al.,[17] and Powell et al.[18]

Melmed reviewed his experience with autologous platelet gel in plastic and reconstructive surgery. He reviewed 53 patients, seven of whom underwent facelifts and 46 of whom underwent breast surgery. Melmed argues that platelet gel is particularly appropriate for patients undergoing procedures that carry a risk of hematoma, specifically facelift, nasal surgery, breast surgery, and skin grafting. Melmed reports advantages including enhanced tissue adhesion, reduction in bleeding, reduction in the risk of bleeding (hematoma formation), promotion of collagenesis, enhanced angiogenesis, increased leukocyte concentration, and the opportunity to avoid the use of surgical drains and nasal packing.

Man et al. presents their experience with 20 consecutive patients, 15 of whom underwent facelifts and five of whom underwent breast surgery. Man et al. advocated the use of platelet gel in procedures associated with capillary bleeding, especially facelift, forehead lift, breast surgery, and abdominoplasty. These investigators noted the advantages of platelet gel as optimizing hemostasis, gluing down flaps, and faster healing. They also highlighted the cost benefit of reducing the use of drains, nasal packing, and bulky dressing materials.

Using fibrin sealant in a double-blind, randomized, controlled trial, Oliver et al.[17] noted significantly less wound drainage, as measured by drain output where fibrin glue was applied to the facial flaps in rhytidectomy. Fibrin sealant imitates the final phase of the coagulation cascade as fibrinogen is converted into fibrin on a tissue surface by the action of thrombin. Fibrin is then cross-linked by factor XIIIa, creating a stable mechanical network of fibrin. This fibrin network seals capillary vessels and allows raw operative surfaces to adhere. The authors noted that a reduction in postoperative drainage could reduce pain and bruising. This obviates the need for drains in facelift surgery, thus creating cost savings.

Powell et al.[18] evaluated the effects of treatment with autologous PRP on postoperative recovery following deep-plane rhytidectomy in a prospective, randomized, controlled study. One side of the face was treated with PRP, while the other side was not. The results were evaluated in a blinded fashion in order to elucidate the effects of PRP in facelift. The authors conclude that treatment with PRP may prevent or lessen edema or ecchymosis after deep-plane rhytidectomy. The trend was more apparent for ecchymosis than edema and was chiefly demonstrable in the early phases of recovery. At first glance, employing a patient as his or her own control would appear to be an elegant experimental model; however, recent evidence suggests that PRP does not create a solely local effect. Rather there may be systemic upregulation,[19] and so the application of PRP to one site may affect healing nearby.

Platelet gel continues to garner interest among facial plastic surgeons because of its ability to reduce infection, swelling, pain, and bruising. Platelet gel purportedly provides the surgeon with hastened wound closure and cosmetically improved suture lines. Other procedures that have been presented and discussed that use platelet gel include laser skin resurfacing, browlift, facelift, rhinoplasty, full- and split-thickness skin grafts, skin flaps, tissue expansion, liposuction, mammoplasty, and other reconstructive procedures.

Indications for Use: A Review of My Clinical Experience

In this discussion I evaluate my experience with autologous preparations of PRP, platelet-poor plasma, and fibrin glue in more than 500 patients undergoing in excess of 1500 facial cosmetic and reconstructive procedures. This experience comprises both major aesthetic procedures including facelift, browlift, blepharoplasty, laser skin resurfacing, and rhinoplasty and minor aesthetic procedures and soft tissue reconstructive cases including local and regional flaps and grafts.

Experience With Platelet-Rich Plasma in CO_2 Laser Skin Resurfacing

My experience suggests that PRP and fibrin glue minimize ecchymosis, reduce edema, and speed healing in facial plastic and reconstructive surgery. However, such variables are difficult to measure as hard endpoints. To evaluate the efficacy of PRP and fibrin glue in wound healing, I carefully examined laser skin resurfacing as an experimental model. In laser skin resurfacing, one may readily measure time to complete re-epithelialization as a hard endpoint, untainted by bias and subjective impressions.[20]

Employing retrospective case-control methods, I reviewed 100 consecutive patients undergoing CO_2 laser skin resurfacing wherein autologous PRP was used during 18 consecutive months. The populations were found to be similar for comparison purposes in terms of age, sex, Glogau scale, Fitzpatrick skin type, and number of passes performed.

The mean blood draw for the procurement of PRP and fibrin glue was 108.8 ml (range: 50 to 188 ml). The subjects were 100 CO_2 laser skin resurfacing patients who underwent 327 concomitant procedures including blepharoplasty (N = 89), facelift or necklift (N = 89), forehead or browlift (N = 18), scar revision (N = 9), chin implant (N = 6), lip fat augmentation or both (N = 5), rhinoplasty or septorhinoplasty (N = 5), chemical peel (N = 4), dermabrasion (N = 1), and scalp reduction (N = 1).

PRP and autologous platelet-poor plasma were procured according to the methods of Perfusion Partners and Associates, Inc. using the Secquire system operated by experienced certified perfusionists. Blood was withdrawn from the patient at the time of surgery (mean: 108.8 ml; range: 50 to 188 ml). Citrate anticoagulant was added to the blood-draw syringe to prevent clotting of the specimen. The blood was subsequently separated into PRP, platelet-poor plasma, and red blood cells. This is accomplished through the centrifugal separation of whole blood during a 12- to 18-minute period.

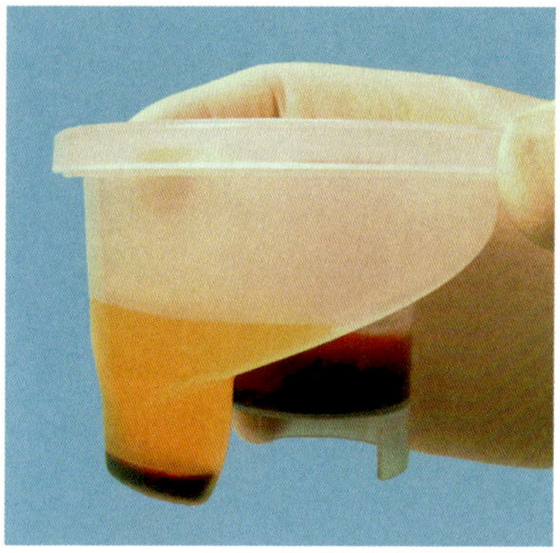

Figure 4-3 The Harvest container after centrifugation of whole blood demonstrates the separation of plasma and platelets from the red blood cells. A platelet-rich pellet is noted at the bottom of the plasma-containing aliquot.

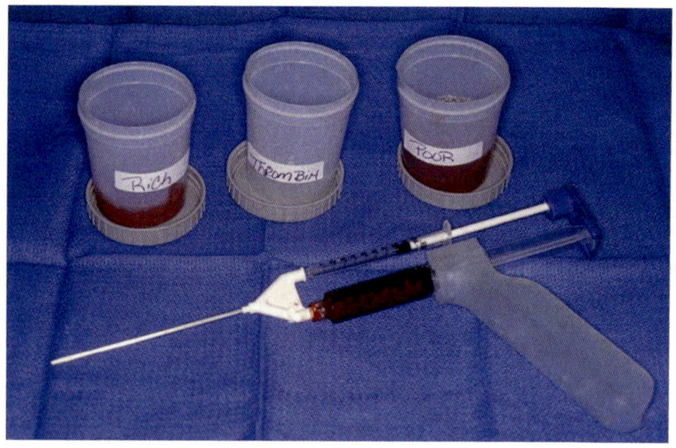

Figure 4-4 Platelet-rich plasma (PRP), platelet-poor plasma, and thrombin are shown on the operative field in specimen containers ready for use. The 10 ml syringe contains PRP and the 1 ml syringe holds bovine thrombin. The dual-tip liquid applicator precisely mixes the PRP and thrombin in a 10:1 ratio.

The PRP comprises approximately 20% of the total blood volume withdrawn from the patient (Fig. 4-3). This solution is used to make the platelet gel and typically represents 10 to 30 ml of the 50 to 188 ml withdrawn from the patient. Once activated with calcified thrombin, within 5 to 30 seconds the platelet-rich solution forms a platelet gel. The activation of PRP or fibrin glue or both is accomplished at the time of surgery through dual-tipped and spray-tip applicators that combine the PRP or platelet-poor plasma with calcium thrombin (1000 U thrombin per 1 ml $CaCl_2$) in a ratio of 10 ml of PRP to 1 ml of calcium thrombin (Fig. 4-4). PRP and platelet-poor plasma may be applied with either a spray or liquid applicator. The applicator allows appropriate mixing and dispensing of the gel and thrombin in a 10:1 ratio precisely and reliably (Fig. 4-5).

Similar proprietary ambulatory systems that enable the rapid, reliable, and simple production of PRP at the time of outpatient aesthetic facial surgery are available from Harvest Technologies and 3I Implant. I have extensive experience with the Harvest system as well as with the Secquire device. Harvest offers two kits. One kit requires 60 ml of blood and yields 7 to 10 ml of PRP and 10 to 20 ml of platelet-poor plasma. The smaller kit uses 20 ml of blood and creates 2.5 to 3.5 ml of PRP and about 5 to 10 ml of platelet-poor plasma (Fig. 4-6).

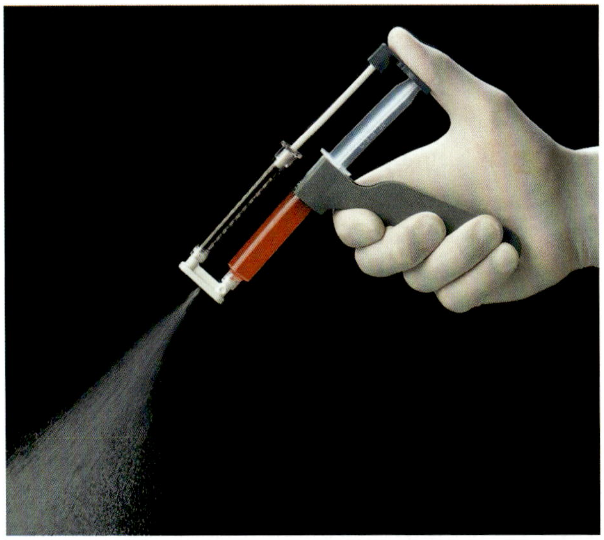

Figure 4-5 The spray-tip applicator creates a fine mist of autologous product.

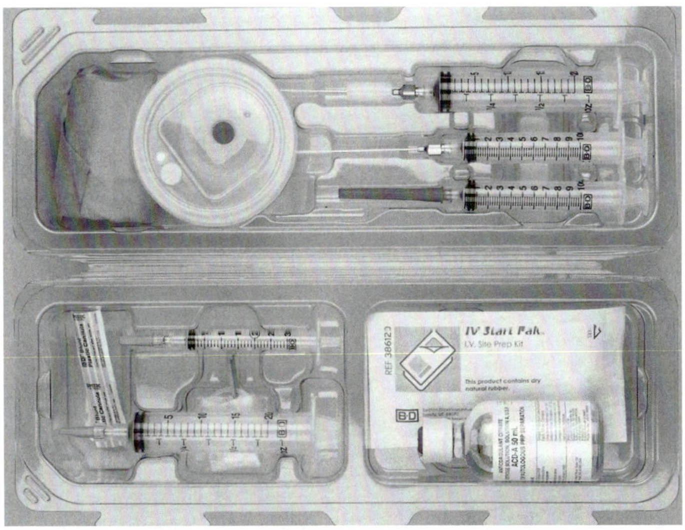

Figure 4-6 The APC-20 kit supplied by Harvest is ready to use with venipuncture supplies and the container for centrifugation and separation of whole blood into platelet-rich and platelet-poor plasma.

In certain regions, independent cardioperfusionists offer mobile platelet gel services to physicians, ambulatory surgical centers, and hospitals. In central Florida, perfusionists charge about \$350 to \$500 per patient for this service. The cost of the disposable items from Harvest and Secquire related to the procurement of PRP is about \$150 to \$250 per patient, but the vendor charges about \$10,000 for the proprietary centrifuge system.

Patients included in the present study with whom I used the Secquire system demonstrated a mean preoperative platelet count of 242,000/μl (range: 145,000 to 386,000/μl). The platelet gel yielded a mean platelet count of 1,200,000/μl with a range of 402,000 to 2,765,000/μl. This represents an increase in platelet concentration of 157% to 1141%. The mean increase in platelet count was 498% ($P < 0.001$, Mann-Whitney U test). I have obtained similar results with the Harvest system.[21,22]

PRP was applied directly to the resurfaced facial skin as a fine mist with the spray applicator. The PRP was allowed to gel, and then platelet-poor plasma was applied over the PRP, creating a gelatin-like mask (Fig. 4-7). Initially, only PRP was applied, but it was noted that the PRP alone tended not to remain in place. Applying the platelet-poor plasma over the PRP created a durable dressing that remained in place until the next morning.

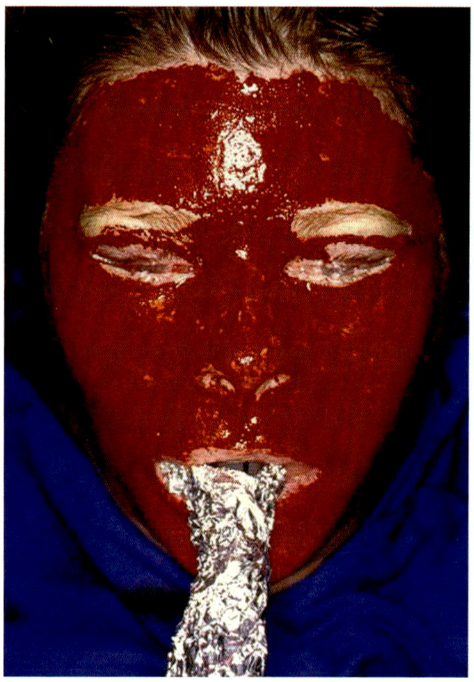

Figure 4-7 Platelet-rich plasma (PRP) is applied directly to the laser-resurfaced facial skin as a fine mist with the spray applicator. PRP is allowed to gel, and then platelet-poor plasma is subsequently applied over the PRP, creating a gelatin-like mask.

To provide a measurable endpoint from which to evaluate the purported advantages of platelet gel, time to re-epithelialization after CO_2 laser skin resurfacing was examined. In the current study, patients undergoing CO_2 laser skin resurfacing (full face or regional) are compared to similarly matched concurrent and historical control patients. The application of platelet gel and fibrin glue was compared with open-technique wound care in laser skin resurfacing. More rapid re-epithelialization of wounds after laser skin resurfacing was observed with PRP. With the application of PRP, the mean time for completion of re-epithelialization was 7.8 ± 2.6 days as compared with 11.4 ± 2.1 days for cases in which PRP was not used ($P < 0.05$; Mann-Whitney U test).

In addition, earlier introduction of makeup was achieved in patients in whom PRP was employed as compared to instances in which open-technique wound care was performed without the application of PRP (9.5 ± 2.2 days vs. 12.8 ± 2.4 days, $P < 0.05$; Mann-Whitney U test). A trend to decreased erythema was noted in cases in which PRP was used as compared with open-technique wound care. A decrease in both duration and intensity of erythema was observed.

Experience With Platelet-Rich Plasma in Deep-Plane Rhytidectomy

The objective of this discussion is to establish the role of PRP and fibrin glue in facial plastic and reconstructive surgery with particular reference to the experience in 65 consecutive facelift procedures during a 12-month period wherein PRP was employed. I perform a deep-plane facelift that typically is accompanied by submentoplasty with suture platysmaplasty. Most facelift procedures are performed with contemporaneous rejuvenative techniques such as subperiosteal midface lift, browlift, blepharoplasty, and laser skin resurfacing.

On completion of the deep-plane dissection technique, excellent pinpoint hemostasis is reassured with careful bipolar cautery. Prior to suture suspension of the composite flap, PRP is applied to the deep plane and subcutaneous dissection to facilitate hemostasis (Fig. 4-8) (2 to 3 ml per side and 1 to 2 ml to the submental region). Suture suspension of the flap is accomplished, and platelet-poor plasma is again applied throughout the subcutaneous dissection plane prior to completing closure (4 to 6 ml per side and 3 to 5 ml to the submental region). The platelet-poor solution is found to optimize hemostasis and facilitate positioning and suspension of the deep-plane composite flap. Multiple layer closure is then accomplished in the usual fashion, and a pressure dressing is applied. Drains may or may not be employed depending on surgeon preference and discretion. In blepharoplasty, a small amount (0.5 ml per lid) of PRP is applied before closure (Fig. 4-9). In browlift, about 2 to 3 ml of PRP is typically employed.

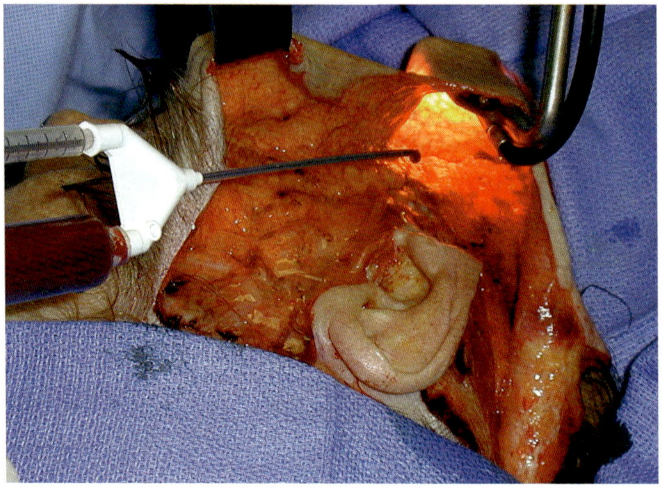

Figure 4-8 Before suture suspension of the composite flap, platelet-rich plasma (PRP) is applied to the deep-plane and subcutaneous dissection to facilitate hemostasis. Approximately 2 to 3 ml of PRP is applied to each side of the face and 1 to 2 ml to the submental region.

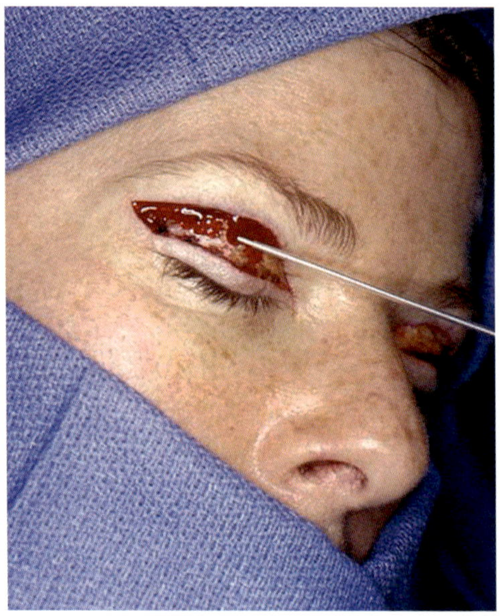

Figure 4-9 In blepharoplasty, a small amount (0.2 to 0.5 ml per lid) of platelet-rich plasma (PRP) is applied prior to closure. In browlift, about 2 to 3 ml of PRP typically is employed.

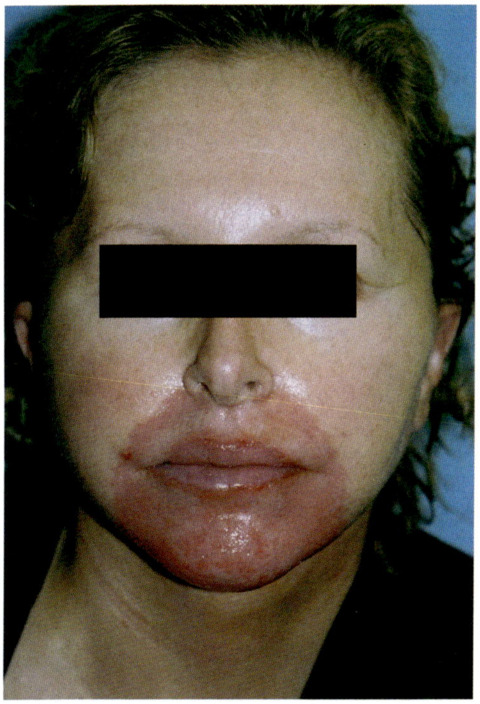

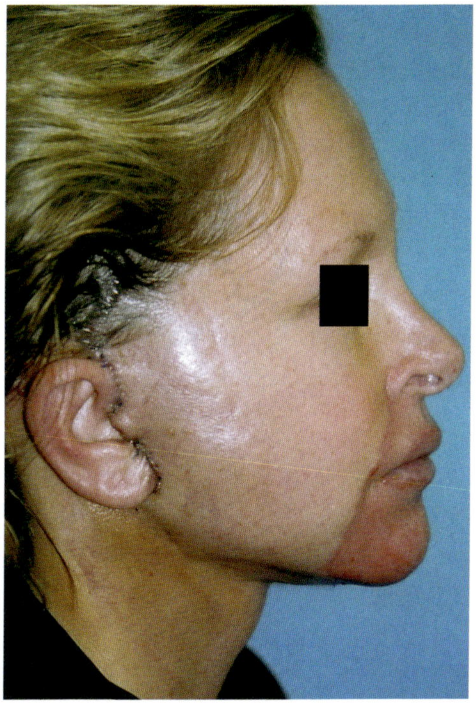

The application of PRP and fibrin glue as described in this discussion appears to speed healing and diminish bruising. The figures above demonstrate the typical postoperative day 1 appearance of a 52-year-old woman who underwent deep-plane facelift with platysmaplasty (and concomitant perioral CO_2 laser skin resurfacing). With the application of PRP and fibrin glue, patients are noted to experience less postoperative pain, as evidenced by the diminished use of postoperative analgesics. Less postoperative steroid use was noted in the experimental group, suggesting diminished or earlier resolution of postoperative swelling and associated discomfort.

In typical facelift surgery without the application of PRP or fibrin glue, I use two Blake drains, one in each hemiface. In facelift surgery with application of PRP and fibrin glue, I have noted that in certain cases the use of drains may be unnecessary. An earlier return to work and activities of daily living is often observed in the PRP group. Because patients treated with PRP and fibrin glue demonstrate shorter recovery times, less intensive perioperative care is required, thus achieving cost savings because of lower utilization rates in terms of number and duration of postoperative office visits. There was no significant difference observed between the two groups in terms of complications, such as hematoma formation.

Contraindications for Use

Contraindications to the use of platelet gel include platelet dysfunction syndromes, critical thrombocytopenia, anemia, hemodynamic instability, and pregnancy. The simultaneous administration of antiplatelet agents and anticoagulants does not generally preclude the successful use of PRP because of the multiple independent pathways of platelet activation; however, the administration of glycoprotein IIB/IIIA inhibitors may impair the effectiveness of PRP because of their activity at the terminal level of platelet activation within the clotting cascade.

Conclusion: Personal Approach to the Use of Platelet-Rich Plasma in My Practice

PRP enhances wound healing. The platelet plays a central role in orchestrating the healing cascade and wound repair process. It follows that increasing the concentration of platelets and their associated signal proteins at the injury site may enhance the healing rate; the application of PRP increases important signal proteins and bioactive molecules at the wound.

Through commercially available ambulatory procurement systems, PRP can safely and efficiently be collected and applied directly to the wound environment in reliably high concentrations in facial plastic and reconstructive surgery. The current chapter suggests that PRP achieves accelerated epidermal and epithelial regeneration with less swelling, more rapid resolution of bruising, and less patient discomfort. These factors translate into less patient down time, earlier introduction of makeup, and earlier return to work.

Laser-resurfaced wounds re-epithelialize more quickly. There was a trend toward decreased duration and intensity of erythema after CO_2 laser skin resurfacing. In facelift and other incisional procedures, benefits also include decreased intraoperative bleeding and the subsequent decreased utilization of postoperative surgical drains and dressings. Less intraoperative bleeding is observed, and so unipolar and bipolar cauterization is reduced, which may induce less trauma and diminish postoperative pain and swelling.

During the course of the study in which platelet gel and fibrin glue were employed, there was a decrease in the use of postoperative surgical drains and dressing materials. Whereas drains were typically employed in facelift surgery in which platelet gel was not used, in cases in which platelet gel and fibrin glue were used, drains were often not employed and less bulky postoperative dressings could be used. The decrease in drain utilization and the application of lighter dressings carries a cost benefit as well as enhanced patient postoperative comfort. Finally, as far as cost benefit is concerned, the more rapid re-epithelialization noted in laser skin resurfacing and the more rapid healing noted in facelift, forehead lift, and blepharoplasty has led to fewer postoperative visits and less intensive postoperative care, thus saving personnel-related costs and physician time.

Autologous platelet gel provides adhesive and hemostatic properties and supplies the wound with growth factors and cytokines that enhance and promote the healing process. In facial plastic surgery, postoperative swelling and ecchymosis are decreased. Cost benefits are recognized through the minimization of drain and bulky dressing use. Personnel costs are also minimized through expedited recovery of the patient, often requiring fewer postoperative visits.

Platelet gel represents an opportunity to optimize wound healing in patients undergoing facial plastic and reconstructive surgery. In addition to major aesthetic surgery, I use PRP in reconstructive and minor aesthetic procedures including local and regional flaps, grafts, lip advancement and augmentation, soft tissue grafts and implants, and dermabrasion and scar revision. Autologous platelet gel significantly minimizes bruising, decreases postoperative pain, speeds healing, enhances flap and graft survival, and hastens re-epithelialization in laser skin resurfacing. Centrifugal methods reliably achieve at least a fourfold concentration in platelets and associated cytokines over baseline. Patient recovery times are reduced 25% to 40%. Patient approval levels are high. Autologous PRP is an important adjunct to acceleration of healing and speed of recovery in patients undergoing facial plastic and reconstructive surgery.

Summary of Key Points

1. PRP is a concentration of platelets and native concentration of fibrinogen harvested by the centrifugal separation of autologous whole blood.
2. With ambulatory procurement systems, PRP can safely and efficiently be collected and applied directly to the wound environment in reliably high concentrations in facial plastic and reconstructive surgery.
3. PRP has an array of cytokines and mediators that increase recollagenation, accelerate epidermal and epithelial regeneration, promote angiogenesis, enhance wound strength, hasten hemostasis, improve tissue regeneration, decrease dermal scarring, and facilitate remodeling.
4. PRP significantly minimizes bruising, decreases postoperative pain, speeds healing, enhances flap and graft survival, and hastens wound re-epithelialization.

REFERENCES

1. Tortora G, Grabowski S. Principles of Anatomy and Physiology, 7th ed. New York: Harper Collins, 1993.
2. Hood AG, Hill AG, Reeder GD, et al. Perioperative autologous sequestration III: A new physiologic glue with wound healing properties. Proc Am Acad Cardiovasc Perfusion 14:126-129, 1993.

3. Kevy SV, Jacobson MS. An automated cost-effective methodology for the preparation of growth factor enriched autologous platelet gel. Presented at the Fourth Annual Orthopaedic Tissue Engineering Meeting, Boston, April 2000.
4. Kevy S, Jacobson M, Benoit PK. The biology of platelet concentrate as prepared by the Harvest Technologies SmartPReP system. Presented at the Third Annual Techvest Conference on Tissue Repair, Replacement and Regeneration, New York, October 23, 2001.
5. Byrne DJ, Hardy J, Wood RAB, et al. Effect of fibrin glues on the mechanical properties of healing wounds. Br J Surg 78:841, 1991.
6. Slater M, Patava J, Kingham K, et al. Involvement of platelets in stimulating osteogenic activity. J Orthop Res 32:263-268, 1993.
7. Marx RE. Platelet-rich plasma (PRP): What is PRP and what is not PRP? Implant Dentistry 10:225-228, 2001.
8. Man D, Plosker H. Discussion: A prospective randomized double-blind trial of the use of fibrin sealant for facelifts. Plast Reconstr Surg 108:2106-2107, 2001.
9. Morita Y, Nishii O, Kido M, et al. Parvovirus infection after laparoscopic hysterectomy using fibrin glue hemostasis. Obstet Gynecol 95:1026, 2000.
10. Wilson SM, Pell P, Donegan EA. HIV-1 transmission following the use of cryoprecipitated fibrinogen as gel/adhesive. Transfusion 31(8S):51S, 1991.
11. Marx RE, Carlson ER, Eichstaedt RM, et al. Platelet rich plasma: Growth factor enhancement for bone grafts. Oral Surg Oral Med Oral Pathol 85:638-646, 1998.
12. Monteleone K, Marx R, Ghurani R. Healing enhancement of skin graft donor sites with platelet-rich plasma. Presented at the 82nd Annual Academy of Oral and Maxillofacial Surgery, San Francisco, September 22, 2000.
13. Kerner MM. The use of autologous platelet-gel as an intranasal dressing in functional endoscopic surgery. Presented at the American Rhinologic Society Meeting, Denver, September 8, 2001.
14. Welsh W. Platelet gel usage in cosmetic surgery. Presented at the American Academy of Cosmetic Surgery 16th Annual Scientific Meeting, Orlando, Fla, January 27-30, 2000.
15. Melmed EP. Autologous platelet gel and plastic surgery. J Aesthetic Surg 21:377-379, 2001.
16. Man D, Plosker H, Winland-Brown JE. The use of autologous platelet-rich plasma (platelet gel) and autologous platelet-poor plasma (fibrin glue) in cosmetic surgery. Plast Reconstr Surg 107:229-239, 2001.
17. Oliver DW, Hamilton SA, Figle AA, et al. A prospective randomized double-blind trial of the use of fibrin sealant for facelifts. Plast Reconstr Surg 108:2101-2107, 2001.
18. Powell DM, Chang E, Farrior EH. Recovery from deep plane rhytidectomy following unilateral wound treatment with autologous platelet gel. Arch Facial Plast Surg 3:245-250, 2001.
19. Buza P. Personal communication. The Florida Platelet Gel Symposium, Melbourne, Fla, April 12, 2003.
20. Clevens RA. Autologous platelet rich plasma in facial plastic surgery. Presented at the Eighth International Symposium of Facial Plastic Surgery, New York, May 1-5, 2002.
21. Marx RE, Kevy SV, Jacobson MS. Platelet concentrate preparation in the office setting: A comparison of manual and automated devices. Unpublished Data, Harvest Corp, July-Sept 2001.
22. Kevy SV, Jacobson MS. Platelet concentrate preparation in the office setting: A comparison of manual and automated devices—Update. Unpublished Data, Harvest Corp, March 2002.

PART II

APPLICATIONS

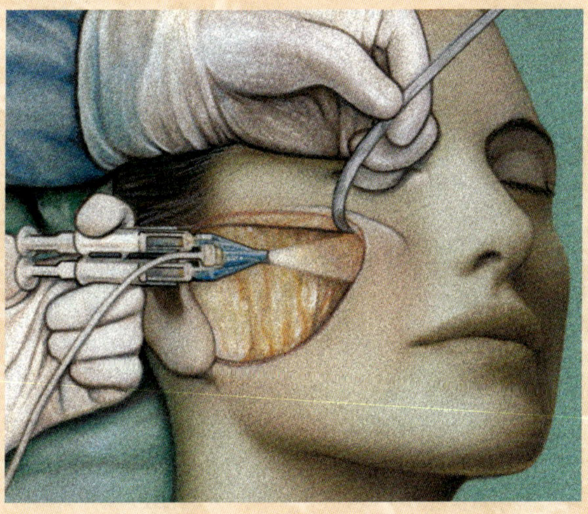

CHAPTER

5

USE OF SURGICAL TISSUE ADHESIVES IN FACIAL PLASTIC SURGERY

Dean M. Toriumi, M.D. ▪ Kevin O'Grady, B.A., B.S.

Technologic advances in instrumentation and biomaterials have increased the efficiency and effectiveness of many of the procedures performed by facial plastic surgeons. With the growing trend to minimally invasive surgery, these technologic developments have enabled surgeons to perform complex surgeries through smaller incisions, with less dissection, less postoperative morbidity, and faster recovery. Surgical tissue adhesives are one class of biomaterials that has proven useful in many surgical specialties. Two main types of tissue adhesives presently are being used in surgery: fibrin-based adhesives and cyanoacrylate tissue adhesives. In this chapter we will discuss the benefits of using these biomaterials and provide insight into how one can maximize their efficacy when used in facial plastic and reconstructive surgery.

Fibrin Tissue Adhesives

Fibrin-based adhesives are derived from the extraction of two naturally occurring plasma proteins, fibrinogen and thrombin, from blood. Fibrinogen, in the presence of thrombin, calcium chloride, and factor XIII, is polymerized into a semisolid fibrin clot useful as an adhesive, sealant, hemostatic agent, and occasionally as a carrier for antibiotics and growth factors.

The strength of a fibrin tissue adhesive is dictated by its fibrinogen concentration. The higher the concentration of fibrinogen, the greater the bonding strength of the adhesive. Similarly the rate at which the fibrin clot polymerizes depends on the thrombin concentration being used. With high thrombin concentration (500 U/ml or greater), polymerization of the fibrin clot is rapid.[1] Rapid polymerization is often desired in cases in which fibrin-based adhesives are being used as either a hemostatic agent or sealant. Conversely, with a low thrombin concentration (10 to 100 U/ml) the polymerization process is relatively slow. Slow polymerization may be desired when the surgeon needs working time to manipulate tissues prior to clot formation. For instance, a surgeon may need time to position a skin flap following application of the adhesive. In such cases the surgeon should use a low thrombin concentration (10 to 100 U/ml), thereby slowing the polymerization process while gaining working time.

Specific instructions are available on the package insert regarding proper dilution techniques and concentrations. When fibrin tissue adhesive is used in surgery, the factor XIII acts to increase the cross-linking of the fibrin polymer and thus creates a more dense fibrin clot.[2]

Fibrin tissue adhesives are available in several different preparations. Homologous fibrin tissue adhesives with high fibrinogen concentrations (75 to 115 mg/ml) are available off the shelf for use in the operating room. Tisseel (Baxter Corporation, Deerfield, Ill.) and Hemaseel (Haemacure Corporation, Sarasota, Fla.) are two of the more popular homologous fibrin-based tissue adhesives. These preparations are made from pooled blood products from patients who have been screened for blood-borne pathogens. The products' components are vapor heat treated with a patented process that kills viral pathogens. The combination of screening and vapor heat treatment has proven to be effective in eliminating potential contaminants.[3] The commercial products also contain an antifibrinolytic agent. The antifibrinolytic agent slows the process of fibrin clot degradation, allowing the fibrin clot to remain in the wound for a longer time. The homologous products are available in a freeze-dried form and require reconstitution into an aqueous state. The thrombin component is readily soluble in the supplied calcium chloride solution. The protein in the fibrinogen component, however, requires a combination of heat and mixing for 20 minutes following reconstitution to dissolve into solution. Once each of the two components is in solution, they can be placed into a delivery device and should be used within 4 hours.

Choosing the proper applicator for delivery of the fibrin tissue adhesive is critical to the successful use of the product. The two components can be mixed by sequential application, simultaneous application, or spray application. Effective polymerization of the fibrin tissue adhesive requires maximal mixing of the fibrinogen and thrombin components. Efficient mixing of the two components in a spray results in maximal strength of the fibrin adhesive and allows the surgeon to deliver less volume of the adhesive to the surgical field. Previous studies have shown that a thick application of adhesive delivered onto a surgical field may act as a barrier to healing or set up a nidus for infection. Spray applicators are the most effective applicators for delivering a thin layer of adhesive with the greatest amount of component mixing for maximal polymerization. Studies by Sierra et al.[4] have shown that sequential application methods provide the least amount of component mixing and likely provide the least efficient use of the fibrin tissue adhesive. Simultaneous application of the two components through a common tip applicator is more efficient than sequential application but is difficult to deliver in a thin uniform coat and still does not provide maximal mixing. Spray applicators provide the most efficient means of mixing, allow application in a thin layer, and uniformly polymerize the fibrin tissue adhesive. This maximal mixing allows the surgeon to use less volume of fibrin tissue adhesive per unit area and still get a good hemostatic and adhesive effect.

Studies conducted at our institution demonstrated that a thick application of fibrin tissue adhesive to a surgical field can compromise wound healing. In this study by O'Grady et al.,[5] split-thickness skin grafts were elevated along the flanks of pigs. The elevated graft skin was trimmed into four 4 by 4 cm grafts bilaterally and reapplied onto the flank following the application of either a thin or thick layer of fibrin tissue adhesive (Fig. 5-1, *A* through *C*). The thin and thick layers consisted of either a 3 or 6 ml total volume of fibrin tissue adhesive applied to the skin graft recipient site with a spray applicator. Following application of the adhesive, skin grafts were placed over the fibrin tissue adhesive to cover the defect. Skin grafts were fixed into position with staples placed at each corner of the graft to minimize the likelihood of any movement or shifting of the skin grafts. The skin grafts were analyzed for graft survival based on observation of areas of demarcation at 1 week, 2 weeks, and 4 weeks after graft placement. The percentage of skin graft survival was determined. The results showed near complete skin graft survival for the grafts treated with a thin layer of fibrin tissue adhesive (Fig. 5-1, *D*). The grafts placed over a thick layer of fibrin tissue adhesive had a dramatically lower skin graft survival with necrosis primarily in areas of the thickest layer of fibrin tissue adhesive (Fig. 5-1, *E*). This study demonstrated the importance of placing a thin layer of fibrin tissue adhesive to maximize healing of skin grafts. Placement of a thick layer of fibrin tissue adhesive may act as a barrier to healing and slow the process of revascularization. This is critical to the survival of skin grafts, as their survival depends on revascularization from the recipient bed. Placement of a thick layer of fibrin tissue adhesive in an area not influenced by revascularization may not affect healing. For example, if a thick layer of fibrin tissue adhesive is placed over a calvarial bone harvest site, hemostasis can be attained with little effect on healing of the overlying well-vascularized scalp skin. The large fibrin clot, however, could act as a nidus for infection.

Clinical Uses

Fibrin tissue adhesives can be used for hemostasis, fixation of tissues, and sealing. Our experience with fibrin tissue adhesives is primarily in the mode of hemostasis. Fortunately most of our surgeries involve relatively little bleeding, and hemostasis can primarily be controlled with bipolar electrocautery. There are some operations, however, that can result in bleeding and hematoma formation. Patients undergoing aesthetic surgery are concerned about bruising and edema, as these consequences of surgery may prolong the healing process and delay their return to a normal lifestyle. For this reason fibrin tissue adhesives can be helpful in aesthetic surgery practice. Whenever we use homologous fibrin tissue adhesives, we obtain consent from the patient and insure they are aware of the homologous nature of these products.

We routinely use homologous fibrin tissue adhesive in our endoscopic browlifts. The release of the periorbita and conservative division of the procerus and cor-

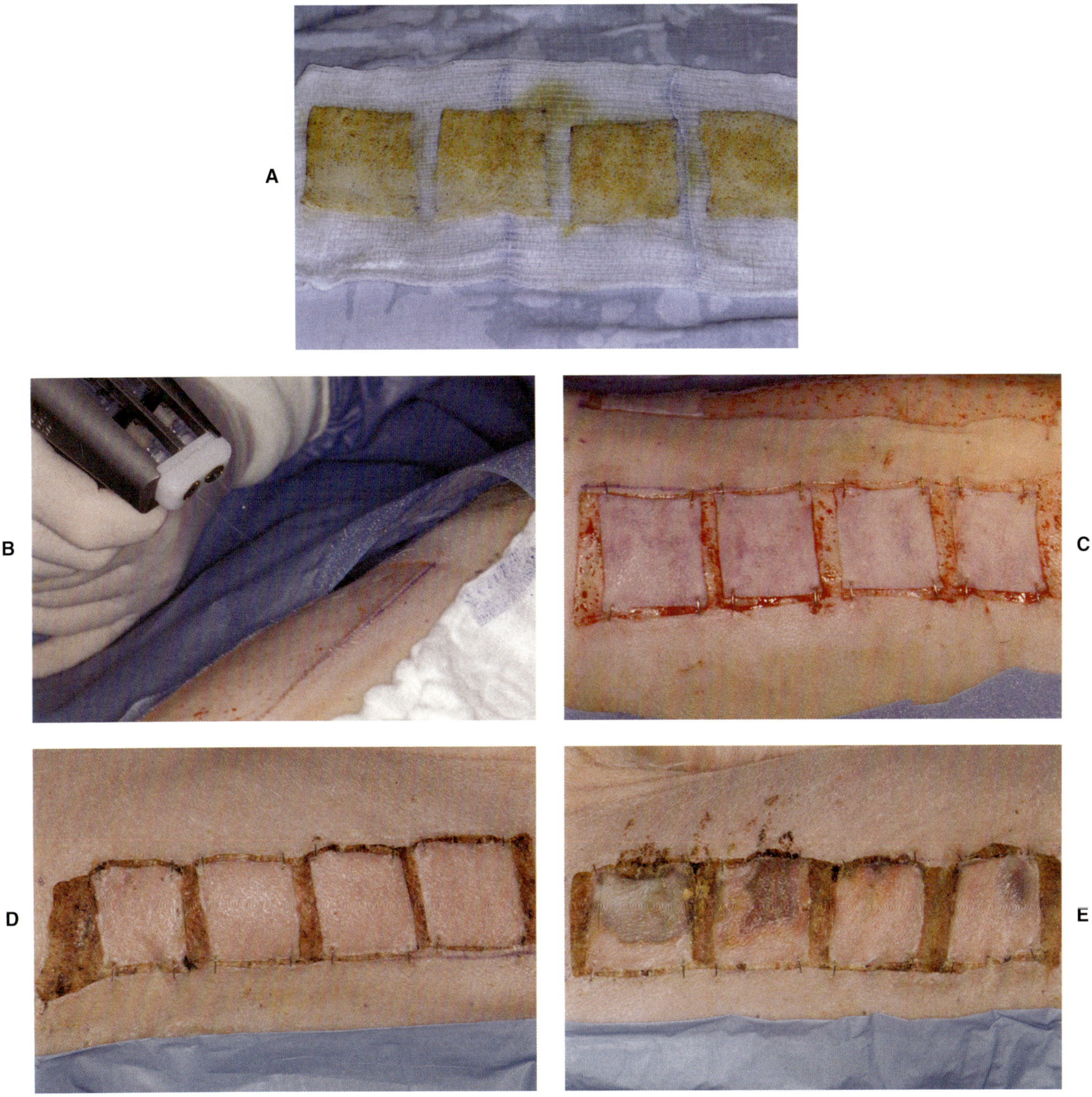

Figure 5-1 **A,** Split-thickness skin harvested from flank of pig and divided into four separate grafts. **B,** Fibrin tissue adhesive sprayed on skin graft site in thin and thick layers. **C,** Skin grafts placed over fibrin tissue adhesive and stapled into position. **D,** Skin grafts over thin layer of fibrin tissue adhesive show excellent skin graft survival. **E,** Skin grafts over thick layer of fibrin tissue adhesive show marked skin graft necrosis.

rugator musculature can result in some bleeding, ecchymosis, and edema. Typically we perform a subperiosteal dissection and a release at the arcus marginalis and then divide the procerus musculature. In a number of cases we will also partially divide the corrugator musculature. After the muscle is divided, we complete the temporal dissection and perform a lateral suture fixation. We usually use bone tunnels for the fixation of the brows; however, the fibrin tissue adhesive can be used for fixation as well. The fixation sutures are placed but not tied until the fibrin tissue adhesive is applied and polymerized. We typically place 2 ml of the homologous fibrin tissue adhesive along the orbital rim and in the midline around the lysed muscles. We use the normal thrombin concentration and apply the fibrin tissue adhesive through a 6-inch (15 cm) malleable, double-barrel applicator tip. This applicator tip can be curved to the proper shape to allow precise application of the fibrin tissue adhesive (Fig. 5-2). After applying the fibrin tissue adhesive, we tie the fixation sutures and then apply pressure to the glabellar region for approximately 5 to 10 minutes. This pressure will allow the fibrin tissue adhesive to polymerize and set with a good bond. Patients treated with the fibrin tissue adhesive have little bruising and edema postoperatively. We have found this use of fibrin tissue adhesive to be beneficial to patient satisfaction (Fig. 5-3).

We also use fibrin tissue adhesives in facelift surgery. We usually use the fibrin tissue adhesive in the cervical region after more extensive neck work or under the skin flaps. The lower fibrin concentration is used to allow extra time to position the skin flaps prior to completion of the polymerization process. We apply the fibrin tissue adhesive with a spray applicator to maximize the use of the fibrin tissue adhesive and make sure that only a thin layer of fibrin tissue adhesive is applied under the skin flaps. Application of too much fibrin tissue adhesive would create a barrier to wound healing and revascularization, which would compromise the viability of the skin flap. We use the lower thrombin concentration to allow more time for positioning of the skin flaps prior to final polymerization. After placement of the fibrin tissue adhesive, pressure is applied for approximately 5 minutes to maximize polymerization. Before the fibrin tissue adhesive is applied, all the flaps are trimmed and then positioned. Key fixation sutures are placed but not tied. Once the fibrin tissue adhesive is applied, the fixation sutures are tied and pressure is applied over the skin flaps. If the skin flaps are moved after the fibrin tissue adhesive is polymerized, the bond between the fibrin clot and the tissues will be disrupted and some of the fibrin polymer effect will be lost. With the use of fibrin tissue adhesive we have eliminated the use of drains.

We also use fibrin tissue adhesives when performing large facial skin flaps for skin cancer reconstruction. In these cases the lower thrombin concentration is used to allow for time to set the facial flaps into position. We trim the skin flap and strategically place fixation sutures to allow the skin flaps to be positioned

A

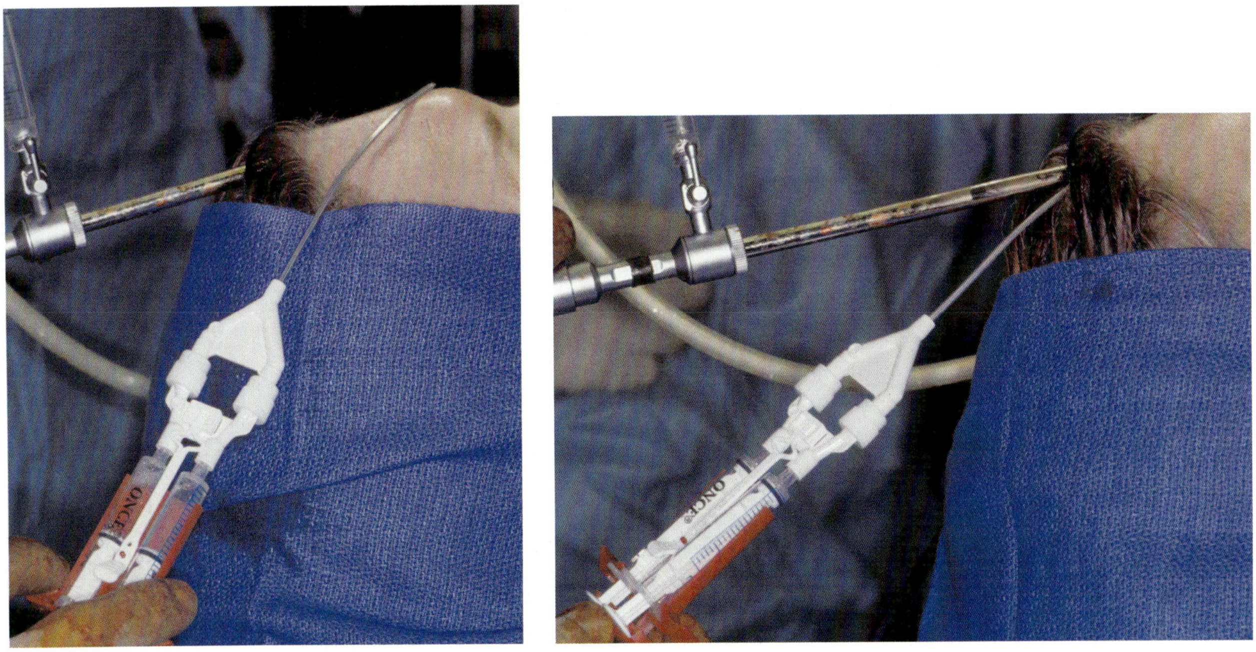

B

Figure 5-2 **A,** Fibrin tissue adhesive is applied with malleable applicator tip under endoscopic visualization. **B,** The applicator tip is advanced to the site of application with slight curvature of the applicator tip.

A

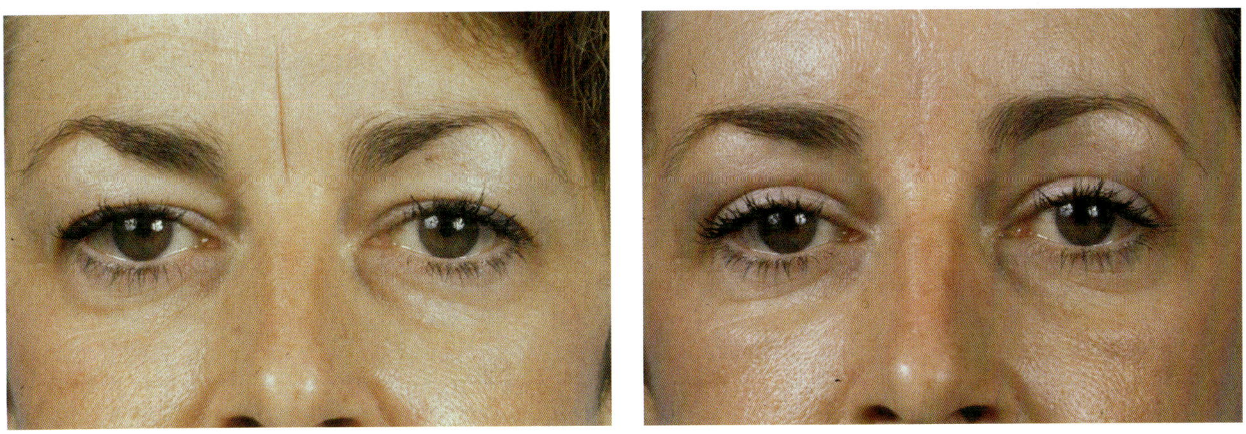

B

Figure 5-3 **A,** Preoperative view of patient with low brows and deep glabellar rhytids. **B,** Postoperative view after endoscopic browlift with lysis of procerus and corrugator musculature. Fibrin tissue adhesive was used to decrease postoperative ecchymosis and edema.

immediately after the fibrin tissue adhesive is sprayed. The fibrin tissue adhesive is sprayed over the area of undermining, and the fixation sutures are tied. Pressure is applied over the surgical site while the fibrin tissue adhesive polymerizes. The fibrin tissue adhesive, even when used for large skin flaps, eliminates the need for drains and decreases postoperative edema and ecchymosis (Fig. 5-4).

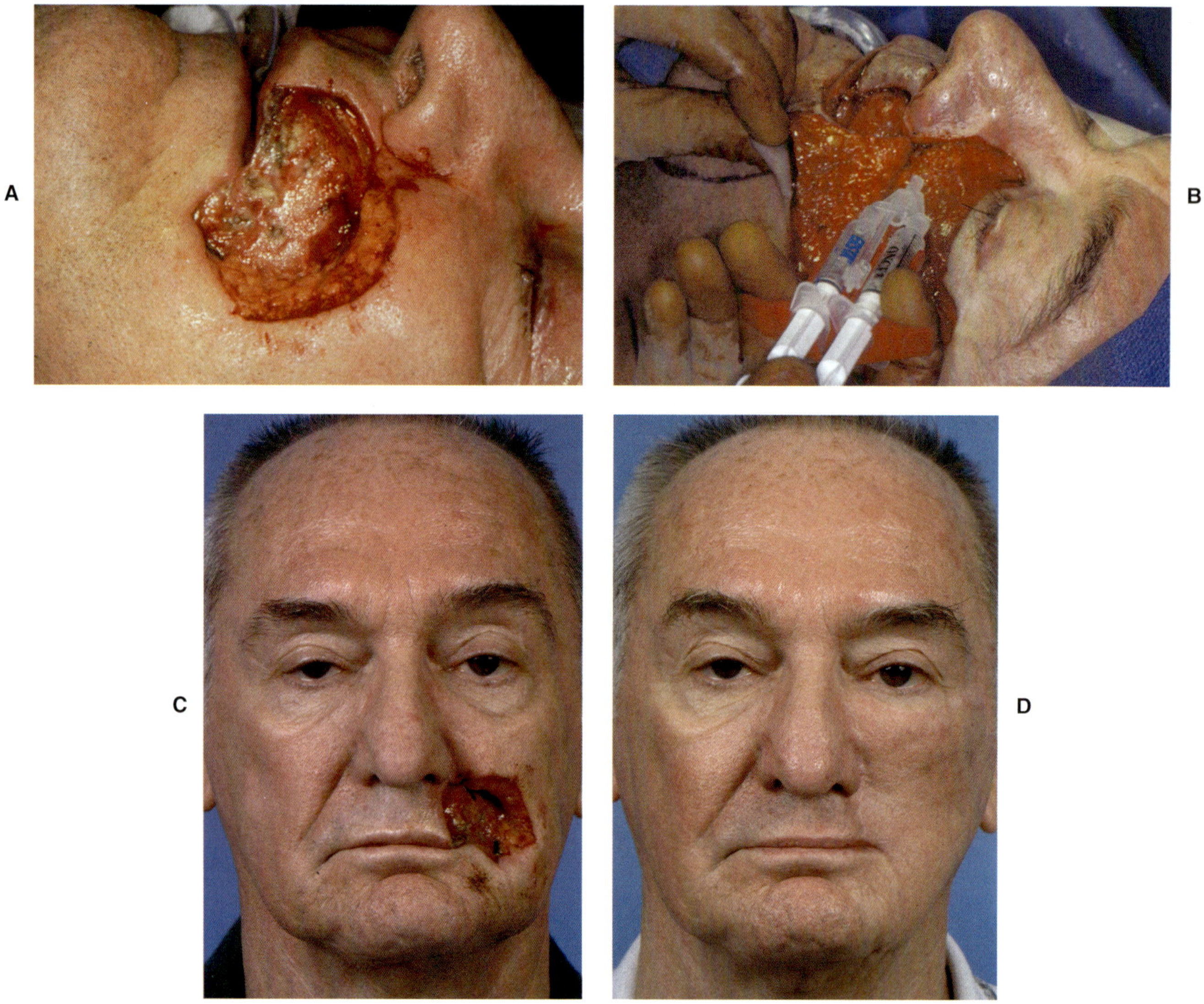

Figure 5-4 **A,** Preoperative defects after Mohs' excision of recurrent squamous cell carcinoma of left cheek and lip. **B,** Application of fibrin tissue adhesive to surgical site. **C,** Preoperative view of Mohs' defect. **D,** Postoperative view after skin flap reconstruction.

PLATELET-RICH PLASMA

A Fibrin-Based Adhesive

Platelet-rich plasma (PRP) is a gel that consists of a high concentration of platelets and a native concentration of fibrinogen harvested by centrifugal separation of autologous whole blood. This platelet concentrate is combined with bovine thrombin to form the gel. It can be made from approximately 70 ml of the patient's own whole blood. Some of the commercially available units are nearly completely automated, allowing more efficient and reproducible platelet recovery and volumes.

The concentration of fibrinogen in PRP is much lower than that in homologous fibrin tissue adhesive. Therefore PRP has much lower tensile strength, or tissue binding strength, and less hemostatic effect. The gel may have a potential to improve healing, but there is little data to substantiate that it improves wound healing in a noncompromised wound. There is, however, a potential that PRP could improve healing in compromised wounds (e.g., chronic, nonhealing wounds, irradiated wounds). Further study will be necessary to determine the true benefit of PRP in wound healing.

Clinical Uses

We use PRP primarily for improving hemostasis in endoscopic browlift and facelift procedures. Patients concerned about use of homologous fibrin tissue adhesives can be offered PRP made from their own blood. Although autologous PRP carries no risk of transmission of an infectious disease, there is a slight risk of factor V cross-reactivity with the bovine thrombin in the PRP. There are discussions in the literature of the risk of antibodies being formed against factor V contaminants in the bovine thrombin.[6] These antibodies have the potential to deplete the patient's own factor V, particularly if the patient had been exposed to bovine thrombin in previous surgery, following which a coagulopathy developed.

Selection of the proper applicator for PRP is important. Spray applicators are preferable, as they will provide better mixing. PRP does not have the same hemostatic and adhesive effects as the homologous fibrin-based adhesives. This will be reflected in the materials' performance. We do not recommend using the PRP for fixation of the brow in endoscopic browlifts, as it does not have sufficient tensile strength to provide adequate fixation.

Cyanoacrylate Tissue Adhesives

Cyanoacrylate tissue adhesives are synthetic adhesives that polymerize in the presence of moisture. They form a bond that is much stronger than the bond seen with fibrin tissue adhesives. When the cyanoacrylate adhesives break down, they form formaldehyde and cyanoacetate. Both of these compounds are tissue toxic. Studies performed in our laboratory demonstrate chronic inflammation after cyanoacrylate is deposited below the level of the skin. In some cases necrosis of tissues was noted.[7] For these reasons, cyanoacrylates should not be deposited subcutaneously and should be limited to applications superficial to the epidermis. Shorter chain cyanoacrylate derivatives degrade at a faster rate and therefore release a larger amount of cyanoacetate and formaldehyde into the tissues over a shorter time. The host is more likely to have an inflammatory response with the shorter chain derivatives. The shorter chain derivatives also tend to be more brittle and may slough off prematurely.

Octyl-2-cyanoacrylate (Dermabond, Ethicon, Somerville, N.J.) was formulated to correct some of the deficiencies of the shorter chain cyanoacrylate derivatives. Octyl-2-cyanoacrylate is an eight-carbon alkyl derivative with a longer carbon chain than the shorter chain cyanoacrylate derivatives (methyl, ethyl, and butyl cyanoacrylate). The longer chain derivative degrades at a slower rate than the shorter chain derivatives do. With the slower degradation rate, tissue inflammation is less should the adhesive inadvertently be deposited below the epidermal level.[8] The octyl-2-cyanoacrylate also contains a plasticizer in its formulation that provides greater pliability than that found in the shorter chain derivatives. The increased pliability allows the material to conform to the site of application and maintain freedom of movement even in areas of maximum tension.

The applicator for the octyl-2-cyanoacrylate has an initiator in the tip, which accelerates the process of polymerization once it is expressed through the applicator tip. During the process of polymerization a small amount of heat is dissipated. If a large volume of monomer is applied to the skin, the heat of polymerization may elicit a burning sensation that could be uncomfortable. It is advisable to apply multiple thin layers of the monomer over the skin. This method of application will decrease the amount of heat dissipated at a given time, and the multiple layers will form a strong, layered adhesive dressing.

A clinical study performed at our institution evaluated the safety and efficacy of octyl-2-cyanoacrylate for closure of incised skin.[9] In this study, 111 patients underwent elective surgical procedures by the same surgeon using either octyl-2-cyanoacrylate or sutures for skin closure. Patients were randomized into either control (vertical mattress suture closure) or test groups (closure with octyl-2-cyanoacrylate). Wounds were evaluated at 5 to 7 and 90 days with the modified Hollander wound evaluation scale. At 1 year, photographs were evaluated by two facial plastic surgeons, who graded the cosmetic outcome using a previously validated visual analog scale. There were no infections or wound dehiscence in either group. Results of the cosmetic evaluations of the scars revealed essentially equivalent outcomes for sutures and octyl-2-cyanoacrylate across all three time periods. This study demonstrated that careful closure of the incisions with subcutaneous suture closure in combination with octyl-2-cyanoacrylate resulted in cosmetic outcomes comparable to suture closure. In this study the special care taken to evert the skin edges with application of the cyanoacrylate adhesive was emphasized and was shown to enhance scar camouflage.

Clinical Uses

Cyanoacrylate tissue adhesives are used exclusively for superficial skin closure. Using a surface adhesive for skin closure is a relatively new concept that requires an approach different from that for traditional suture skin closure. When skin is closed with sutures, the angulation and positioning of the skin suture can act to evert the edges of the wound. When a surface adhesive is used to close skin, however, the biomechanical effect of the suture is lost. In fact there may be a tendency for the skin edges to invert if the cyanoacrylate is not applied properly. One of the keys to successful skin closure, and subsequently to a good aesthetic outcome, is the elimination of subcutaneous dead space. Subcutaneous dead space can be eliminated by placing precise subcutaneous sutures (Fig. 5-5, *A*). Proper placement of subcutaneous sutures will closely approximate the skin edges, closing the dead space, and may act to evert them. A Webster-type everting subcutaneous suture is applied a distance from the skin edges to evert them. To obtain a good aesthetic outcome with cyanoacrylate skin closure, Webster-type subcutaneous sutures should be used to assure skin edge eversion (Fig. 5-5, *B*). Once the subcutaneous dead space is eliminated and the skin edges are closely approximated, the cyanoacrylate adhesive can be used to approximate the epidermal skin edges. We prefer to apply the cyanoacrylate adhesive in small volumes along the incision to "spot weld" the incision closed. It is helpful to use fine forceps to evert the skin edges as the cyanoacrylate adhesive is applied (Fig. 5-5, C). The spot welding application minimizes the likelihood of "gluing" the forceps to the wound. If a moderate amount of skin edge eversion can be accomplished with the cyanoacrylate adhesive, good scar camouflage may be achieved (Fig. 5-5, *D*). On the other hand, if subcutaneous dead space is not eliminated, the scar may invert, creating a depressed scar (Fig. 5-5, *E* and *F*). This inversion of the wound occurs weeks to months after the closure, as scar contracture acts to close the dead space.

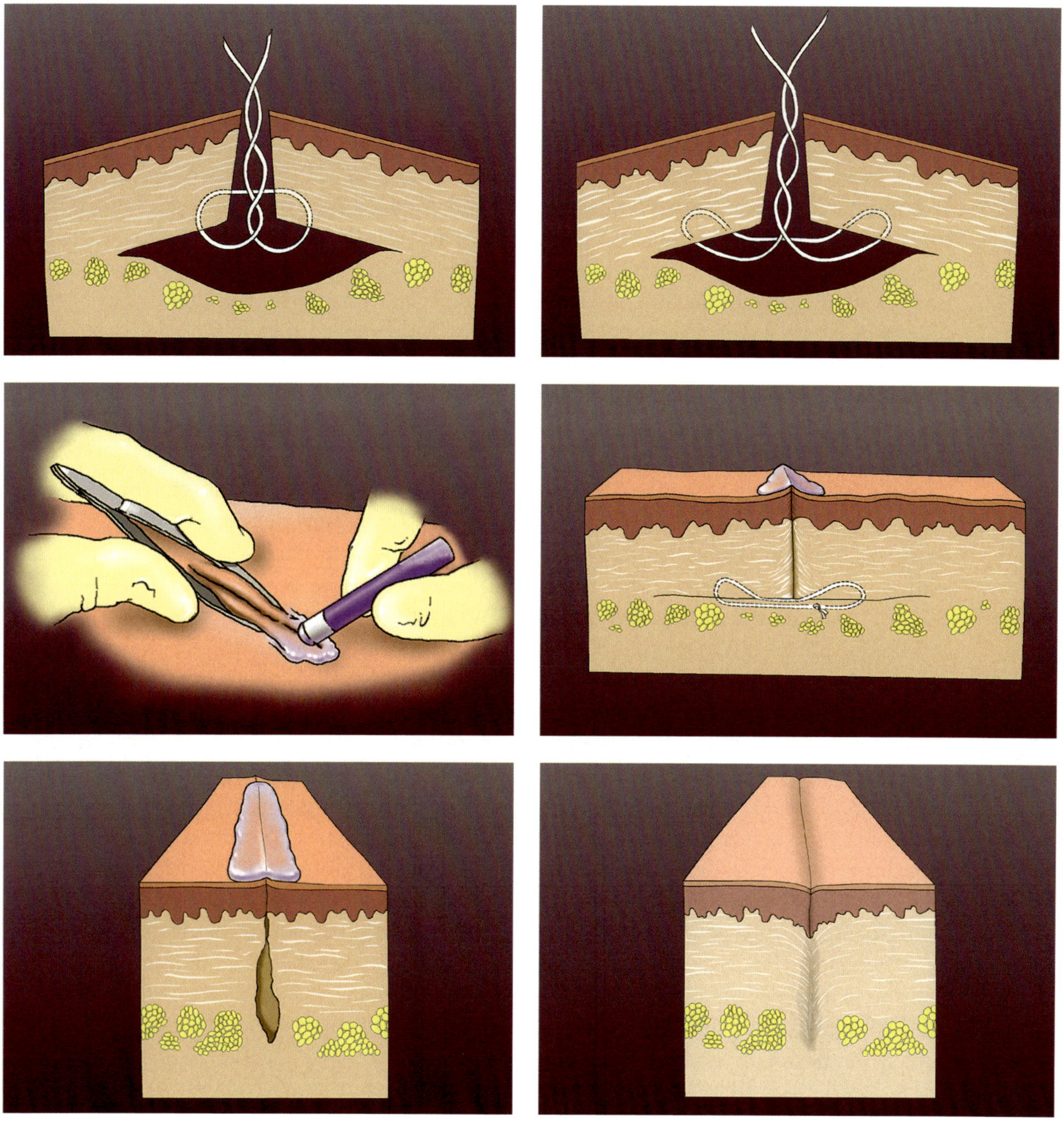

Figure 5-5 **A,** Proper placement of subcutaneous sutures can eliminate subcutaneous dead space and maximize alignment of skin edges. **B,** Webster-type everting subcutaneous sutures are placed beyond the edges of the undermined skin edges and act to hyperevert the skin edges. **C,** Cyanoacrylate adhesive can then be applied to the approximated skin edges with the help of fine forceps. **D,** If adhesive is applied properly, the skin edges will be everted with elimination of the subcutaneous dead space. **E,** It is not advisable to apply cyanoacrylate adhesive to approximate the epidermal skin edges unless the subcutaneous dead space has been eliminated. **F,** If subcutaneous dead space is left below the skin closure, this space will contract and the skin edge may invert leaving a depressed scar. (From Toriumi DM, O'Grady K, Desai D, Bagal A. Use of octyl-2-cyanoacylate for skin closure in facial plastic surgery. Plast Reconstr Surg 102:2209-2219, 1998.)

In some cases a few 6-0 fast-absorbing catgut vertical mattress sutures can be used to approximate and evert the skin edges prior to placement of the cyanoacrylate adhesive (Fig. 5-6). When the cyanoacrylate polymer peels off, the fast-absorbing gut will come off with the polymer adhesive. It is important to avoid depositing cyanoacrylate polymer below the level of the skin. Deposition below the level of the dermis may set up a chronic foreign body giant cell reaction. In most cases the polymer will extrude over time. If the polymer is deposited deep below the skin, it will remain in that position until it is degraded.

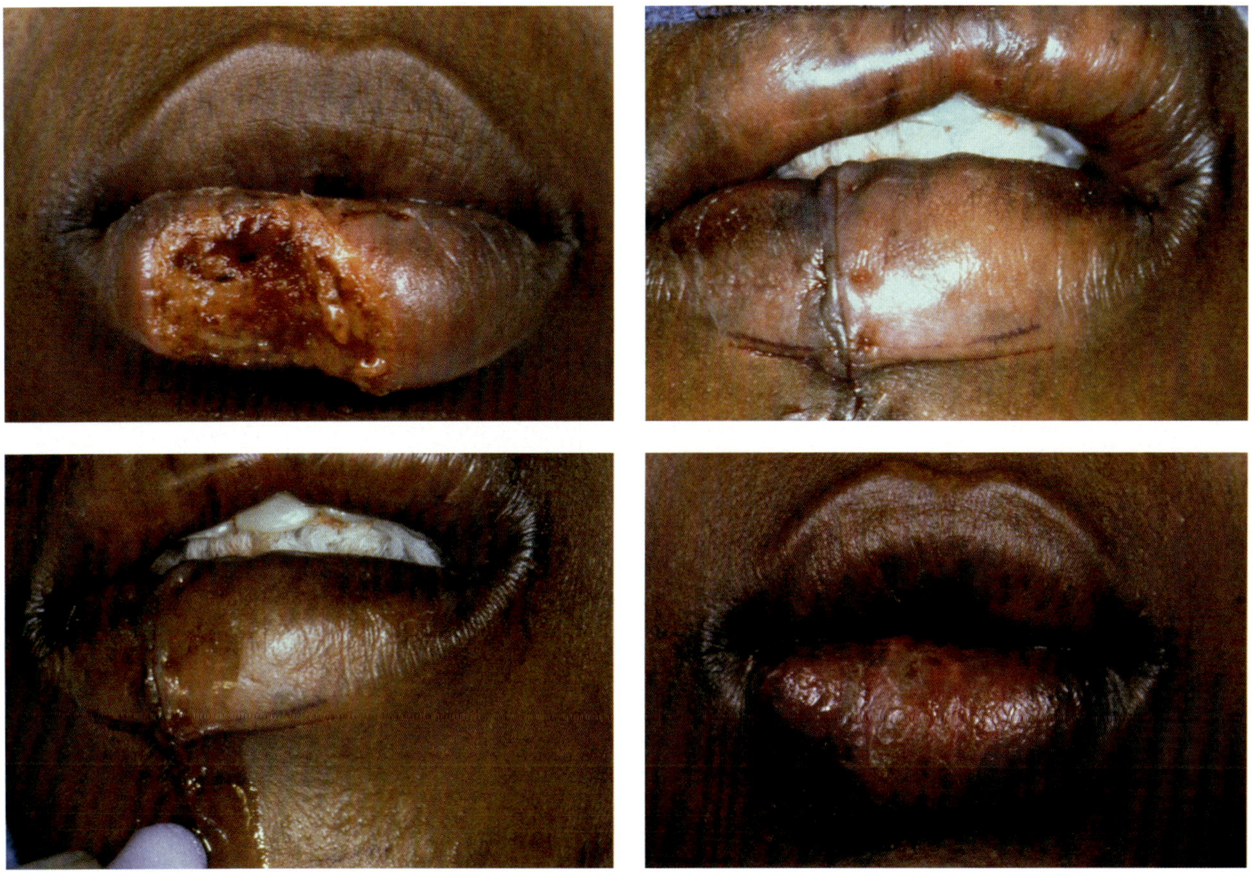

A B C D

Figure 5-6 **A,** This patient suffered a human bite to her lower lip that involved both mucosa and skin. **B,** After waiting for several days for antibiotics to take effect, the wound was closed with subcutaneous 5-0 polydioxanone sutures (PDS) and a few 6-0 fast-absorbing catgut vertical mattress sutures. **C,** The remainder of the closure was accomplished with the cyanoacrylate tissue adhesive. **D,** The incision healed well with little scarring.

When cyanoacrylate adhesive is being applied to an incision, it is preferable to apply it in multiple thin layers. It will take about 2 to 3 minutes to fully polymerize depending on how much monomer is applied. If larger aliquots of monomer are dropped on the wound as it is applied, it may run away from the wound. To better control the monomer, the patient can be positioned so the surgical field is flat or canted so the run off will move away from important structures such as the eyes. If some of the cyanoacrylate should get into the eyes, antibiotic ophthalmic ointment can be applied to the area. Over time the polymer will lift off without damaging the eye. In fact, cyanoacrylate adhesives have been used to treat corneal abrasions. We do not advise this. However, the cyanoacrylate adhesive will not damage the cornea as long as it is not peeled off the cornea. If one is working near the hairline, petroleum ointment can be applied to the hair, and if cyanoacrylate gets into the hair, the petroleum ointment will minimize the adherence of the polymer to the hair follicles (Fig. 5-7).

We have used cyanoacrylate adhesives for closure of many different skin incisions. The cyanoacrylates work well for closure of most facial incisions including, for example, facelift incisions, blepharoplasty incisions, closure of facial defects (see Fig. 5-7), and scar revisions. When using the cyanoacrylates for closure of facelift incisions, we prefer to use 5-0 polydioxanones (PDS) subcutaneous sutures and strategically placed 6-0 fast-absorbing gut vertical mattress sutures followed by the octyl-2-cyanoacrylate for superficial skin closure. The fast-absorbing catgut vertical mattress sutures provide some skin edge eversion and ensure that critical areas of the incision are adequately approximated. In most cases, four or five fast-absorbing catgut vertical mattress sutures are used for each side of the facelift closure. When the cyanoacrylate peels off, the fast-absorbing catgut comes off with the polymer.

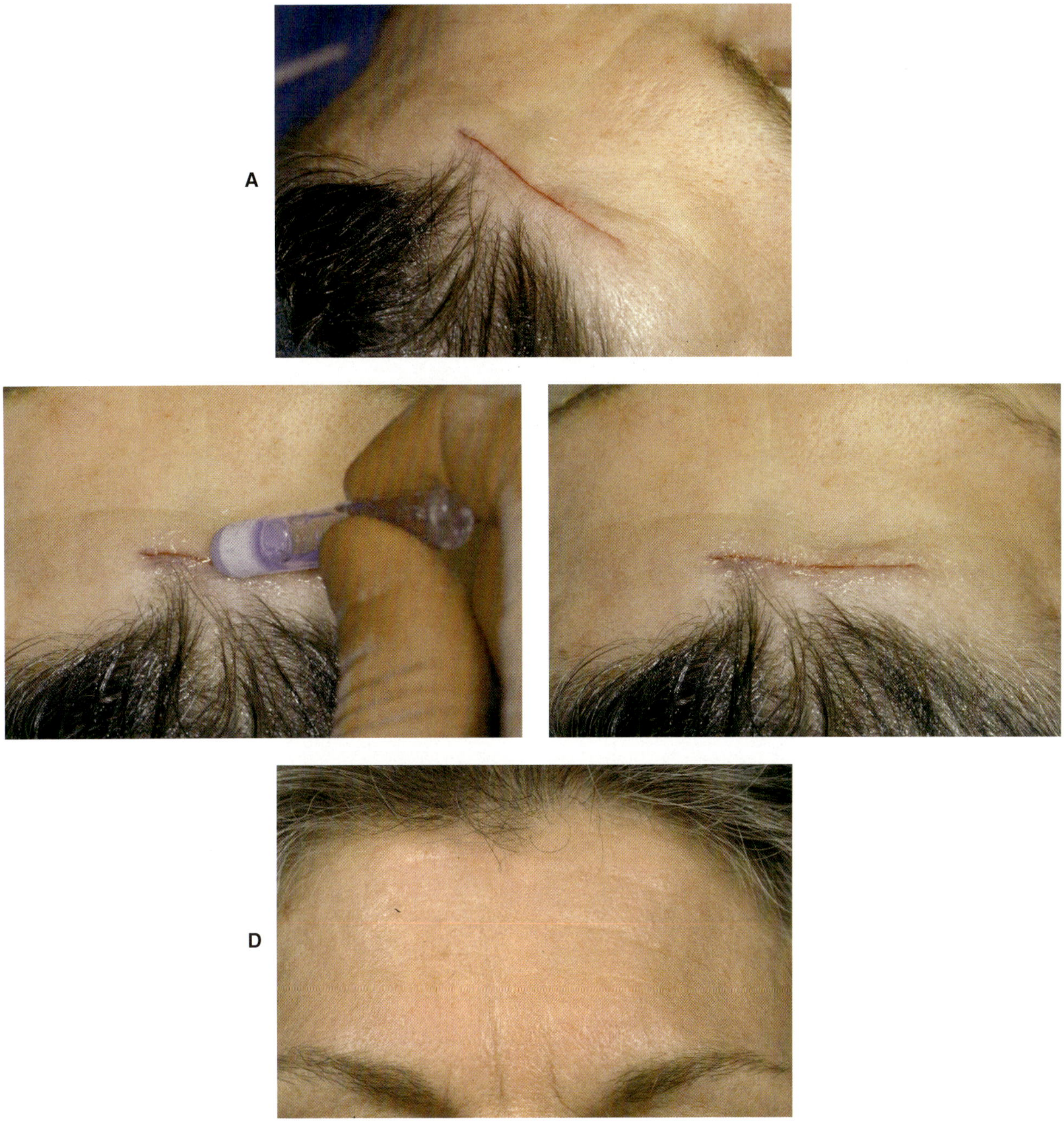

Figure 5-7 Scar following excision of a basal cell carcinoma. **A,** The skin was closed with subcutaneous 5-0 polydioxanone sutures (PDS). **B,** Cyanoacrylate tissue adhesive was applied to the skin edges. **C,** The adhesive is polymerized providing good approximation of the skin edges. Note the hair is protected with ointment to prevent adherence of the polymer to the hair follicles. **D,** Acceptable healing of the scar.

Scar camouflage for facelift incisions is excellent with use of 5-0 PDS subcutaneous closure, 6-0 fast-absorbing catgut vertical mattress sutures, and cyanoacrylate closure of epidermal skin (Figs. 5-8 and 5-9).

A

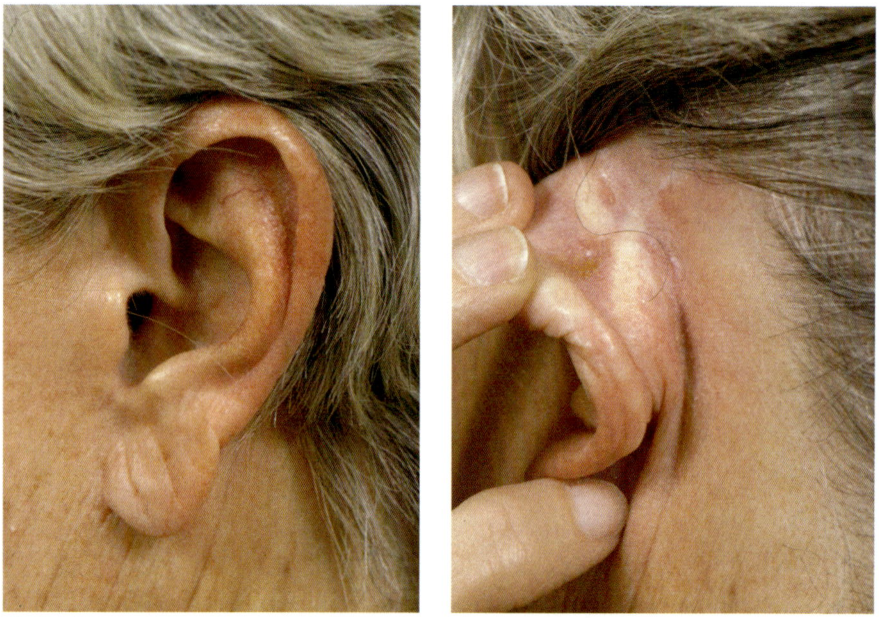

B

Figure 5-8 Facelift incisions closed with cyanoacrylate tissue adhesive. **A,** Preauricular incision. **B,** Postauricular incision.

A B

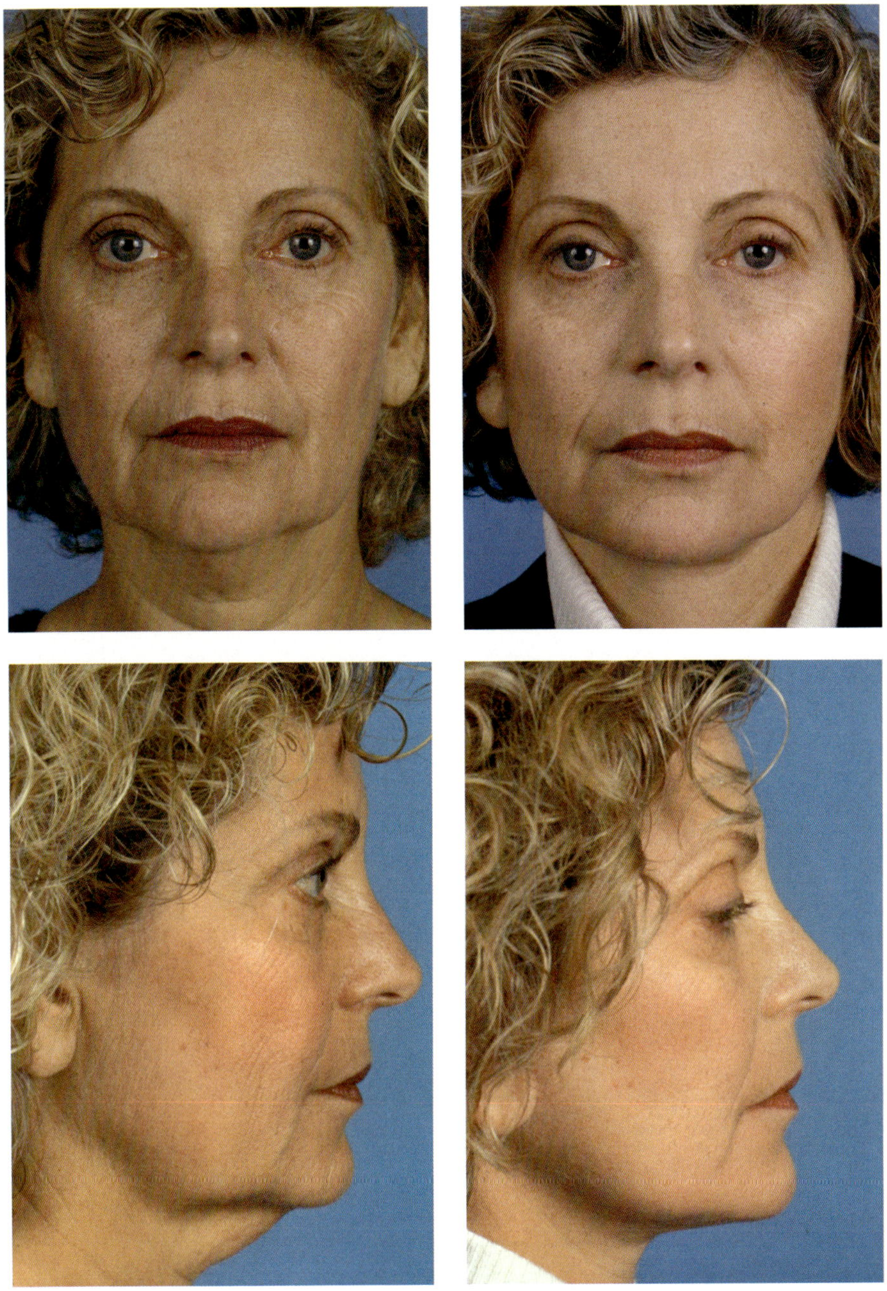

C D

Figure 5-9 Patient undergoing facelift with skin closure using cyanoacrylate tissue adhesive. **A** and **C**, Preoperative views. **B** and **D**, Postoperative views.

For upper blepharoplasty incisions a small volume of cyanoacrylate should be used so that the function of the eyelid is not limited. Two or three 6-0 fast-absorbing catgut sutures will aid in approximating the skin edges and make it easier to complete the closure with the cyanoacrylate adhesive (Figs. 5-10 and 5-11). Special care must be taken in applying the cyanoacrylate adhesive to eyelid incisions to avoid its adherence to eyelashes or the cornea. The octyl-2-cyanoacrylate now comes in a fine applicator tip that will allow a thinner, more controlled application of the monomer. Additionally, the octyl-2-cyanoacrylate comes in a new, more viscous version that will enhance handling and site-specific application of the product (Dermabond). Heat of polymerization is slightly higher with the more viscous octyl-2-cyanoacrylate; therefore thin layers of the adhesive should be applied to allow better dissipation of the heat.

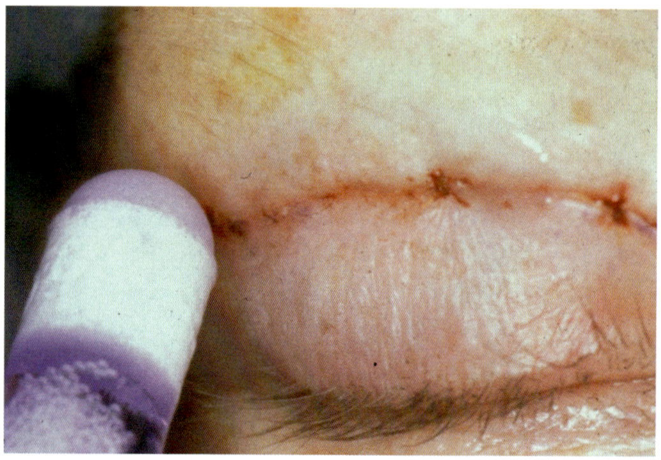

Figure 5-10 A couple of 6-0 fast-absorbing catgut sutures are placed to approximate the skin edges of the upper blepharoplasty incision. The cyanoacrylate adhesive can be applied to the incision to complete the closure.

The primary advantage of using octyl-2-cyanoacrylate for skin closure is eliminating the need for suture removal. For some patients suture removal is traumatic, and elimination of this process can be important to them. This is particularly true in patients undergoing cosmetic surgery. Additionally, facelift patients may have numerous sutures in tender areas, where their removal causes much discomfort. With simple removal of the cyanoacrylate polymer at about 10 days after surgery, the incision will be well healed and the patient will not experience any painful suture removal.

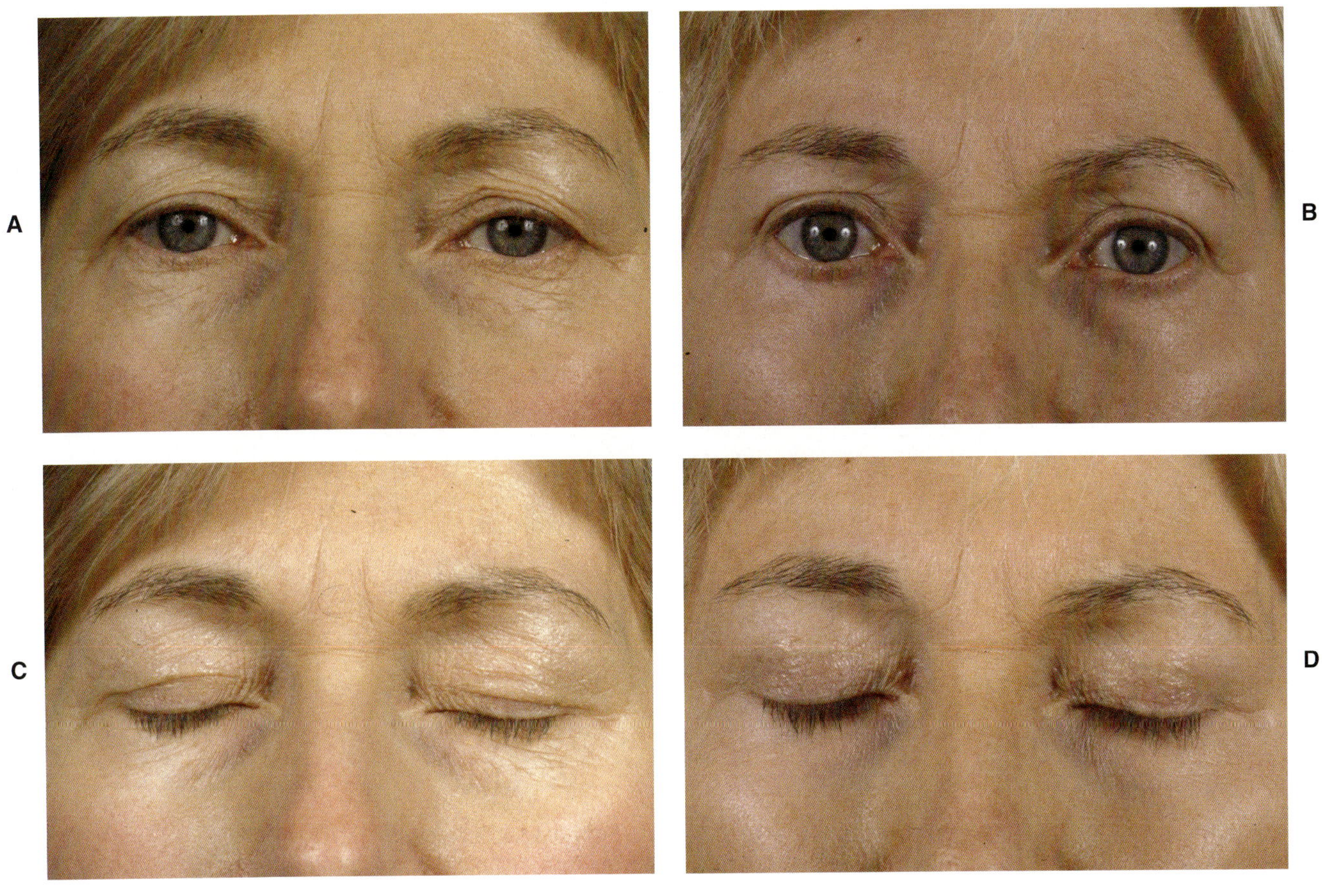

Figure 5-11 Patient underwent upper blepharoplasty and closure of the skin edges with cyanoacrylate tissue adhesive. Note how the upper eyelid incision is well healed. **A** and **C,** Preoperative views. **B** and **D,** Postoperative views at 1 year.

Octyl-2-cyanoacrylate is particularly advantageous in the pediatric patient. In these patients suture removal can be difficult and traumatic (Fig. 5-12). The octyl-2-cyanoacrylate is also useful for patients who are not mobile, have difficulty keeping office visits because of travel constraints, or live a great distance from the surgeon's office.

A B

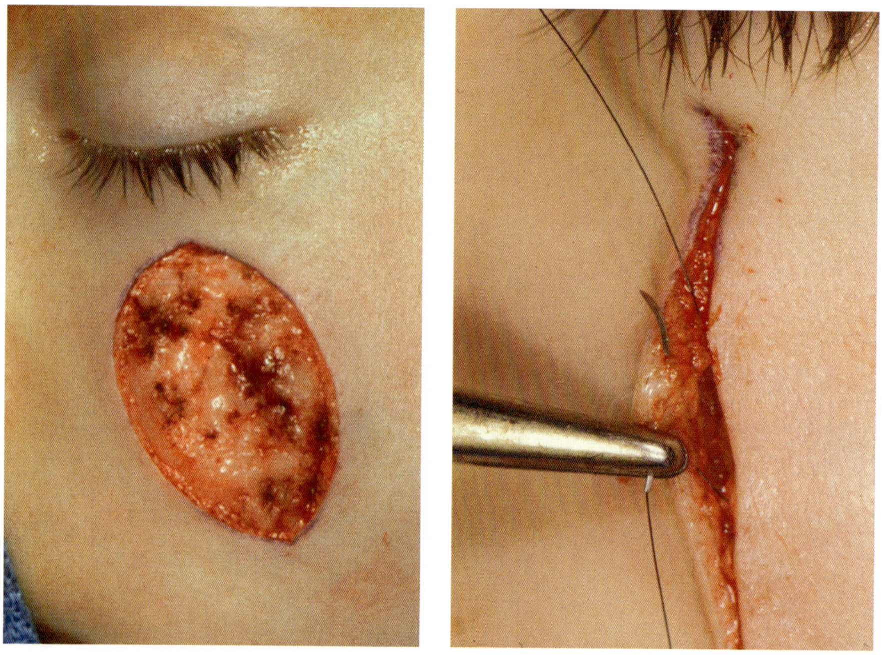

Figure 5-12 **A,** Pediatric patient with defect after excision of giant hairy cell nevus. **B,** Subcutaneous 5-0 polydioxanone sutures (PDS) were used as well as a running 5-0 Prolene intradermal suture to approximate the epidermal skin edges.

C D

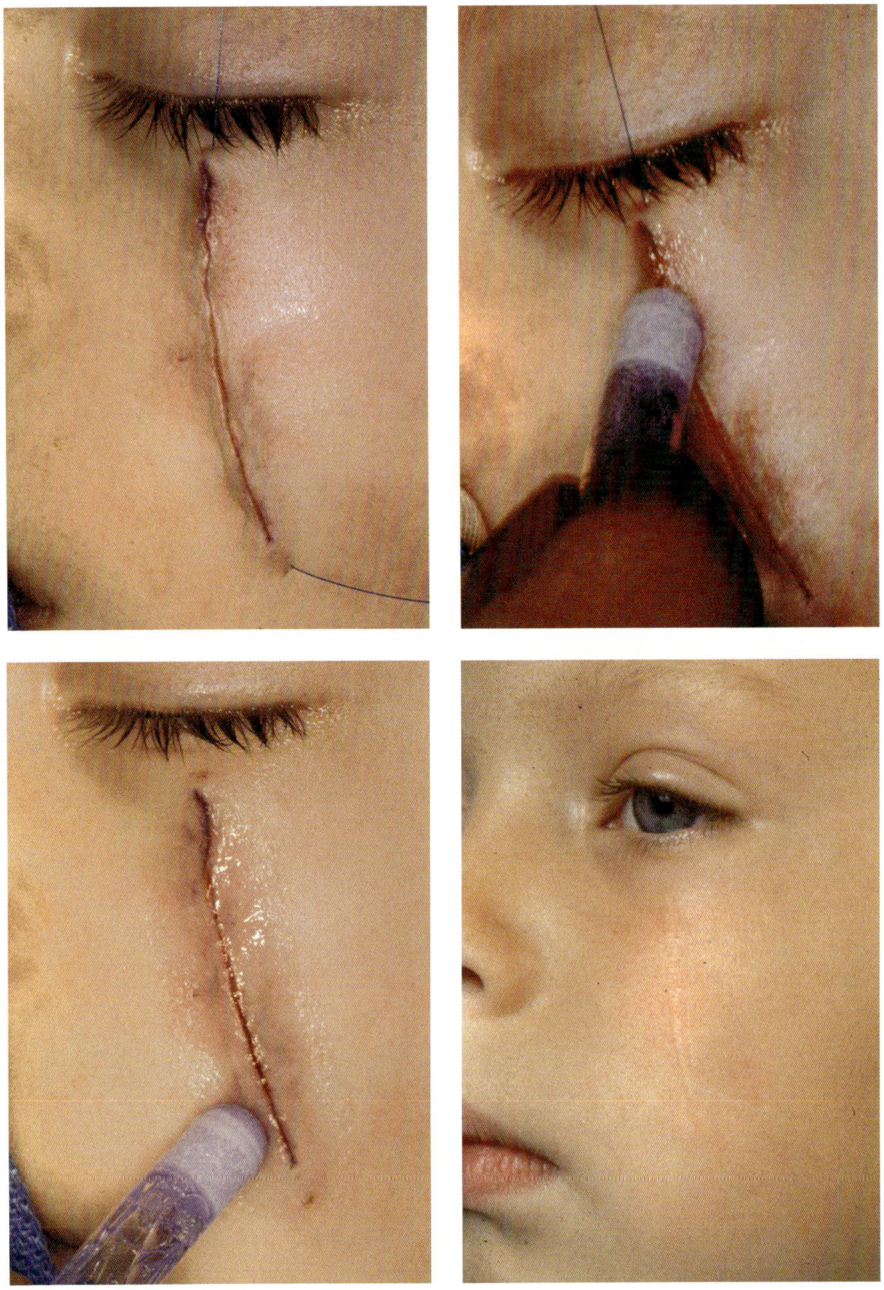

E F

Figure 5-12, cont'd **C,** The skin edges are approximated. **D,** Skin closure is completed with cyanoacrylate adhesive. **E,** The Prolene suture is removed after the cyanoacrylate is polymerized. The Prolene suture was temporary to closely approximate the epidermal skin edges. **F,** Postoperative result with acceptable outcome at 1 year.

Additionally, ocytyl-2-cyanoacrylate can decrease operative time for procedures that require complex skin closures. Numerous sutures may be required to close complex scar revisions, such as Z-plasties, geometric broken line closures, or W-plasties. In cases such as these, skin closure time can be decreased substantially through the use of octyl-2-cyanoacrylate (Fig. 5-13).

To achieve results with octyl-2-cyanoacrylate comparable to those with sutures, the surgeon must take special care in executing the incision precisely and eliminating subcutaneous dead space by placing subcutaneous sutures. The subcu-

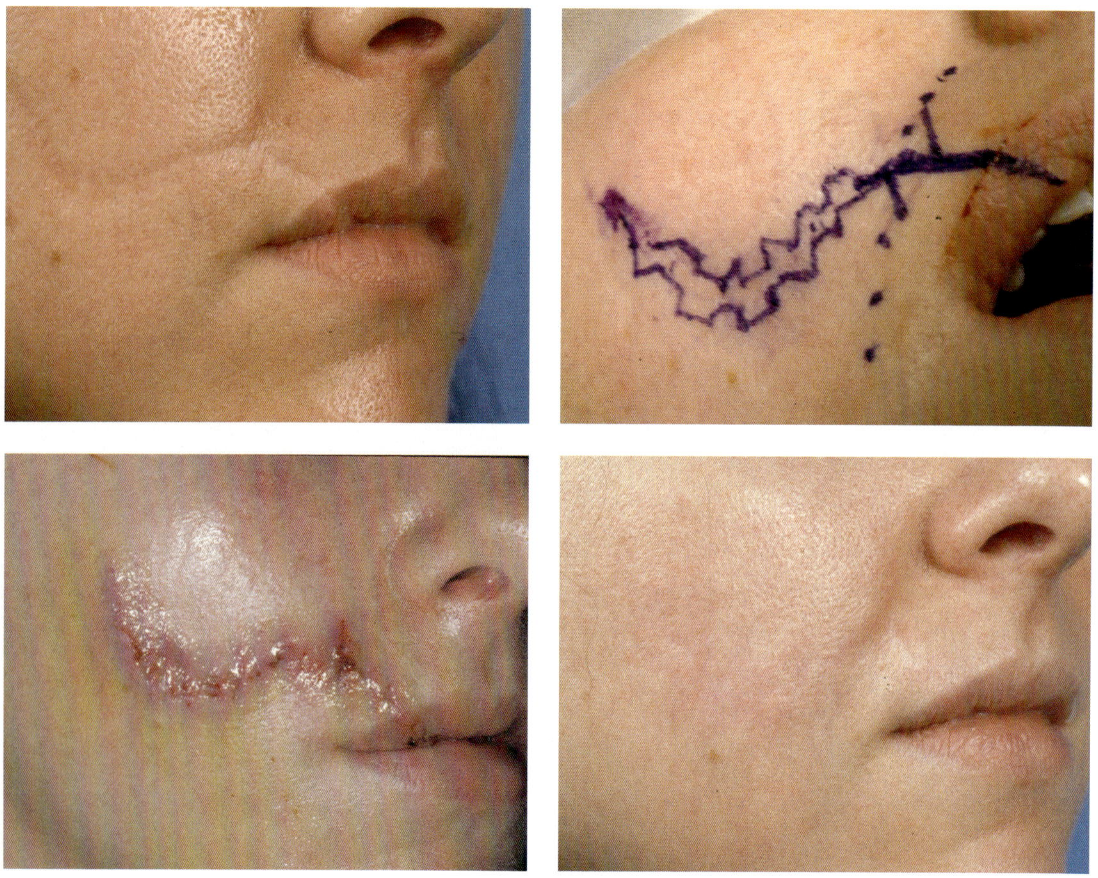
A B C D

Figure 5-13 **A,** Patient with a large scar on her cheek from an automobile accident. **B,** Planned out geometric broken line closure and Z-plasty at the cheek lip fold. **C,** Octyl-2-cyanoacrylate used to close the epidermis after subcutaneous 5-0 polydioxanone sutures (PDS) have been placed. The octyl-2-cyanoacrylate significantly shortened the time to complete the skin closure. **D,** Postoperative result showing acceptable scar camouflage at 2 years.

taneous sutures should provide a moderate degree of skin edge eversion prior to placement of the octyl-2-cyanoacrylate. Fine-tooth forceps can be used to aid in skin edge approximation at the time of application of the cyanoacrylate adhesive. In many cases, strategically placed 6-0 fast-absorbing catgut vertical mattress sutures can be used to better approximate the skin edges before the epidermal closure is completed with the cyanoacrylate adhesive. Cyanoacrylate adhesives are ideal for use in cosmetic surgery to decrease the time involved in skin closure and to minimize discomfort associated with suture removal.

Final Comments

Surgical tissue adhesives can be helpful in facial plastic surgery. Fibrin tissue adhesives are used primarily for hemostasis and fixation of tissues. Minimizing postoperative ecchymosis and edema allows patients undergoing aesthetic facial surgery to return to normal work-related and social activities in a shorter time. The octyl-2-cyanoacrylate can be used for superficial skin closure. This adhesive can eliminate the need for superficial sutures and suture removal. This is particularly helpful in patients undergoing cosmetic surgery, in pediatric patients, and in patients who are particularly bothered by suture removal. In many cases fibrin tissue adhesives can be used in combination with octyl-2-cyanoacrylate, as both adhesives have different properties. We frequently apply the fibrin tissue adhesive below the level of the skin closure for hemostasis and apply the octyl-2-cyanoacrylate for superficial skin closure.

References

1. Hermans J, McDonagh J. Fibrin: Structure and interactions. Semin Thromb Hemost 8: 11-24, 1982.
2. Redl H, Seelich T, Guttman J, Dinges H, Schlag G, Kuderna H, Stachelberger H. Basic Considerations and Theoretical Background of Fibrin Sealing. Presented at the Fourteenth Congress of the European Society for Surgical Research, Barcelona 1979.
3. Radosevich M, Goubran HA, Burnouf T. Fibrin sealant: Scientific rationale, production methods, properties, and current clinical use. Vox Sang 72:133-143, 1997.
4. Sierra DH, O'Grady KM, Toriumi DM, Foresman PA, Rodeheaver GT, Eberhardt A, Feldman DS, Lemons JE. Effects of mixing on fibrin sealant mechanical properties. J Biomed Mater Res 52:534-542, 2000.
5. O'Grady KM, Agrawal A, Bhattacharyya TK, Shah A, Toriumi DM. An evaluation of fibrin tissue adhesive concentration and application thickness on skin graft survival. Laryngoscope 110:1931-1935, 2000.
6. Nichols W. Adverse antibody-mediated reactions to topical bovine thrombin and fibrin glue. Symposium on Fibrin Sealant: Characteristics and Clinical Use. Bethesda, Uniformed Services University of the Health Sciences, 1994, pp 5-10.
7. Toriumi DM, Raslan WF, Friedman M, Tardy ME. Histotoxicity of cyanoacrylate tissue adhesives: A comparative study. Arch Otolaryngol Head Neck Surg 116:564-550, 1990.
8. Leonard F, Kulkarni RK, Brandes G, et al. Synthesis and degradation of poly (alkyl alpha-cyanoacrylates). J Appl Polymer Sci 10:259, 1966.
9. Toriumi DM, O'Grady K, Desai D, Bagal A. Use of octyl-2-cyanoacylate for skin closure in facial plastic surgery. Plast Reconstr Surg 102:2209-2219, 1998.

CHAPTER

6

Use of Fibrin Sealant in Endoscopic Browlift

Daniel Marchac, M.D. ▪ Santiago Goni, M.D.

Plastic surgeons were quite late in discovering the possibilities of endoscopy in facial surgery. It was Vasconez et al.[1] and Isse[2] who first used it for frontal rejuvenation, and that remains its major application.

Our experience with frontal endoscopy began in 1993 after we visited Nicanor Isse. We have used the endoscope 16 times for removal of various lesions at the forehead level, such as dermoid cysts, steel wires protruding after frontal remodelings, and osteomas, with excellent results. But results of endoscopy for aesthetic correction of the forehead have been especially positive, and we have performed 668 cases of frontal endoscopy since 1993. This technique has totally replaced the coronal frontal lift in our practice. Unlike most surgeons, we use fibrin glue for fixation rather than any of the various suspension methods using screws and sutures.

We have used fibrin glue in many surgical procedures, including skin grafts,[3] nerve repair,[4] craniofacial surgery,[5] and aesthetic surgery.[6] Its use improves hemostasis of raw surfaces, obliterates dead space, and permits a closer apposition of healing tissues. In rhytidectomies the use of fibrin glue has decreased the incidence of hematoma and reduced postoperative edema and ecchymosis, obviating the need for postoperative dressings.[7] Nevertheless, we now tend to limit the use of sprayed fibrin glue in facelifts only to selected patients with oozing or unstable blood pressure.

In endoscopic forehead lifts, once the appropriate soft tissue work has been performed, the issue of repositioning the undermined forehead must be resolved. Since there is no scalp resection with the endoscopic technique, one must use an alternate method for maintaining the desired position postoperatively until a fibrous adhesion forms. The senior author (D.M.) has used fibrin glue for facelifts and bicoronal forehead lifts since 1983[8] with satisfactory results. It was thus chosen as our method of fixation for endoscopic forehead lifts (Tissucol, Baxter-Immuno AG, Vienna, Austria).

We present the experience of nearly 700 procedures performed by D.M. in which he used fibrin glue for isolated endoscopic forehead rejuvenation procedures, often associated with blepharoplasties or cervicofacial lifts.

Patient Evaluation

Before surgery, the patient is asked to frown and elevate the eyebrows to assess for the desired postoperative positioning, and photographs of the patients are taken at rest, while frowning, and while elevating the eyebrows. The strength of the corregator and frontalis muscles is rated from 1 (minimum) to 4 (maximum). The skin excess between the eyebrows, the vertical excess at the root of the nose, and the horizontal wrinkles are also evaluated. We measure the distance between the eyebrows as well and evaluate their horizontal position by measuring the vertical distance between the inner portion of the eyebrow to the inner canthus, to the pupil, and to the external canthus. These measurements will enable comparison with the postoperative results.

Preparation of Material

The fibrin glue is prepared when surgery is ready to begin. Generally 2 ml is used. When the eyebrows must be elevated significantly, we use 4 ml. A special long cannula for depositing fibrin glue in deep wounds is used to distribute the mixture of fibrin glue and thrombin on the forehead.

Timing in Use of Materials

Once the forehead has been elevated under the periosteum, the periosteum along the supraorbital rim has been transected, and the muscle has been cut, the extent of eyebrow mobilization is again checked, and then quickly the fibrin glue–thrombin combination is injected with the long cannula. The forehead is then immobilized for 40 seconds with the hands.

Preparation of Wound

The forehead is approached through four openings: two temporal and two paramedial. The two temporal incisions correspond to the end of our horizontal temporal incision for the facelift approach. If the endobrow is done without facelift, we place the horizontal incision at the same level, in view of the future facelift. The two paramedial incisions are made transversely 3 cm apart. When we first began to do endoscopic forehead lifts, we made the two paramedial incisions vertically, but some scars were noticeable because the hair was parted vertically. We have no problems now because we use a 1 cm transverse scar. The hair is not shaved, and the transverse incision is performed down to the bone. A Tegaderm (3M, Minneapolis, Minn.) dressing is placed on the hair, which is combed, sometimes with a gel if it is curly, and the incision is made through the Tegaderm over the previous scalp incisions.

Technique

Intravenous sedation with propofol allows painless injection of lidocaine combined with epinephrine at 1% concentration. The supraorbital region and areas to be incised are especially infiltrated. If a significant elevation is planned or if the hairline is placed quite high, a more liberal injection with 0.5% lidocaine is used.

Four incisions are used for the approach: two temporal and two paramedian. When the forehead lift is performed in association with a cervicofacial lift (which is most cases), the anterior part of the temporal incision is used. When the frontal lift is an isolated procedure, we place the 1.5 cm horizontal incision at the same level.

Medially, two short incisions are placed transversely, 4 cm apart, 1 cm behind the hairline. The left one (for the scope) is 0.8 cm long, and the right one (for the instrument) is 1.2 cm long.

The dissection starts laterally using Mayo scissors to undermine the temporal region and freeing the aponeurosis from the temporal crest to enter under the periosteum of the forehead, from the side toward the middle (lateral to median). A special long elevator is then used to raise the periosteum from the bone, up to the hairline and down to the supraorbital rim. The same maneuver is performed on the other side. The medial part of the periosteal elevation is performed from the paramedial incisions with great care, striving to be as even as possible and not to rupture the periosteum.

Posteriorly the periosteal elevation is performed in proportion to the planned elevation of the eyebrows, stopping at the hairline when no significant elevation of the eyebrows is planned and going as far back as the top of the head if a significant elevation of the eyebrows is desired.

A large occlusive Tegaderm dressing is placed over the paramedian incisions to stabilize the hair and keep the operative area clean. The endoscope (40 mm, 30-degree angle) and the elevator are introduced through the Tegaderm dressing glued on the combed hair (Fig. 6-1, *A*).

Elevation of the periosteum to the supraorbital rim is completed under endoscopic control. The periosteum is then incised transversely at the level of the supraorbital rim, as low as possible, with the elevator or with a semicutting curved hook (Fig. 6-1, *B*) (Pouret Medical, Clichy, France). The neurovascular pedicles and corrugator and procerus muscles become visible and are identified (Fig. 6-1, C).

The procerus muscle will then be transected at the root of the nose with the semicutting hook, which will sever the muscles and preserve vessels and nerves (Fig. 6-1, *D* and *E*). The corrugator muscles are resected with a cutting grasper if quite thick or with the curved hook if thin. The nerves and vessels are carefully preserved; small bleeding veins are coagulated if necessary.

A 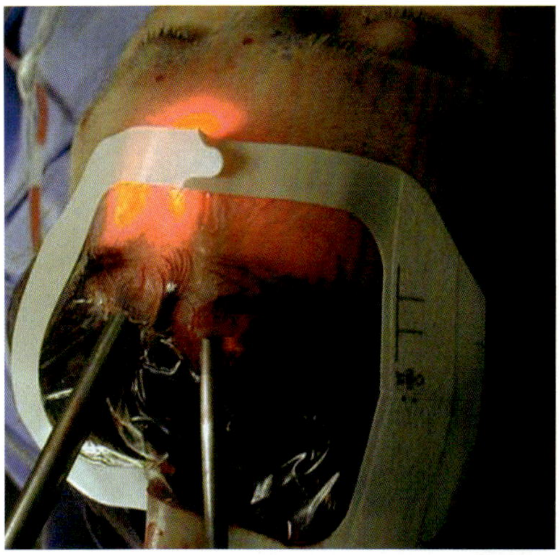

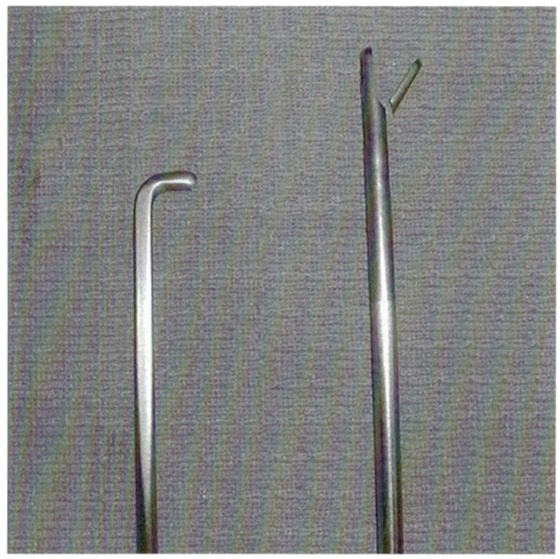 B

C 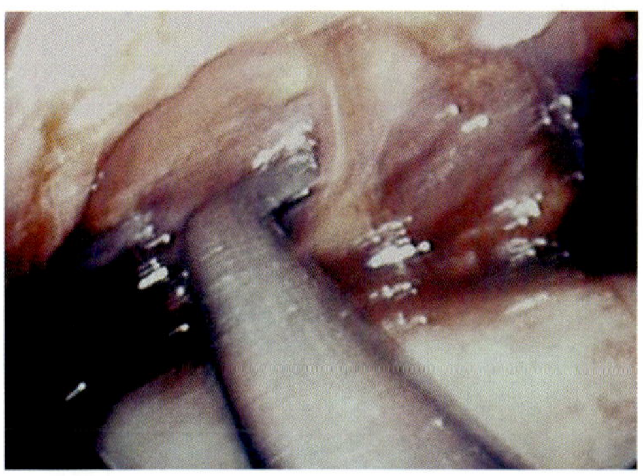

Figure 6-1 **A,** Incision through plastic sheet; insertion of scope *(left)* and elevator *(right)*. **B,** Semicutting hook *(left)* and cutting grasper *(right)*. **C,** The curved hook dissects the supraorbital pedicle. **D** and **E,** The semicutting hook cuts the periosteum and the muscles **(D),** not the nerves and vessels **(E).**

D 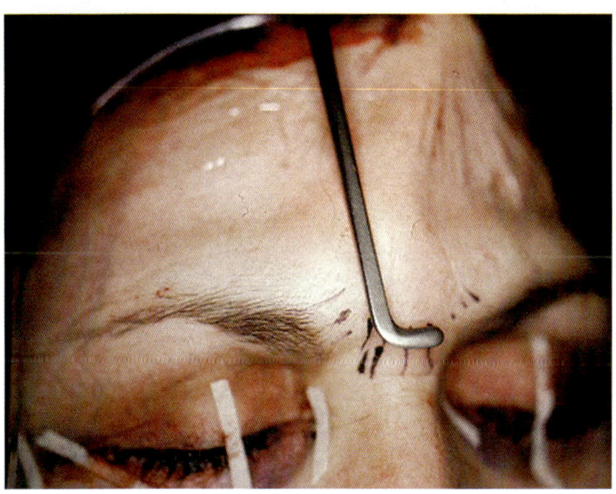

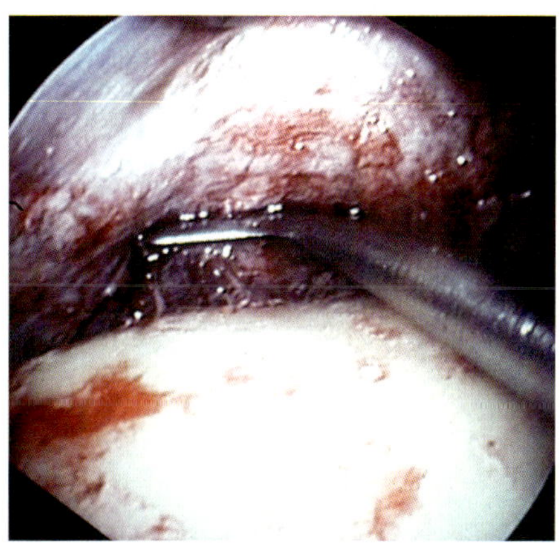 E

The periosteum from the supralateral angle of the orbit is then visualized and, if necessary, is carefully elevated, being certain to remain as close to the bone as possible to avoid injury to the frontal branch of the facial nerve. The periosteum, along with the lower insertion of the frontalis muscle, is cut completely. One should see the yellowish subcutaneous tissue of the upper eyelid.

Sometimes when there is a deep glabellar wrinkle, an incision is made through the periosteum at the upper level of the wrinkle, which is identified with a needle. A subcutaneous tunnel is made with endoscopic scissors down to the lower end of the wrinkle. A fragment of periosteum or a dermal strip (from facelift skin resection) is introduced in the tunnel to fill the wrinkle.

Fixation With Tissue Glue

One should check that the brows and soft tissue move freely and symmetrically before the fixation is performed. With a long cannula a mixture of fibrin and thrombin is distributed in the undermined areas through all four incisions. When only a minor elevation is needed, 2 ml is sufficient, and 4 ml is needed when a significant elevation is planned (Fig. 6-2, A).

The desired position of the forehead skin, as was determined before the operation, is obtained through a combination of transverse spreading and a variable degree of elevation. When there is severe sagging of the eyebrows, the subperiosteal undermining must be extended behind the hairline, and elevation of the forehead creates some recession of the hairline. In most cases the required elevation is minimal, and the hairline will not be displaced because the fixation is done mostly in the lower part of the forehead.

A

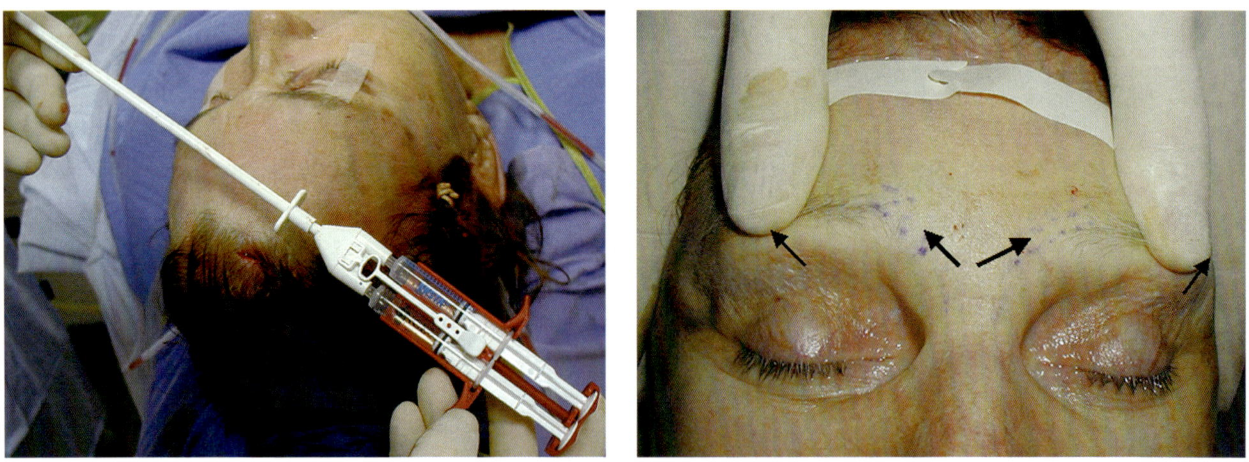

B

Figure 6-2 **A,** Fixation by spreading 2 ml of fibrin glue. **B,** Desired position (generally, moderate elevation and spreading) is maintained for 40 seconds.

The gluing allows selective positioning with (1) spreading of the glabellar area and medial elevation, (2) lateral elevation and spreading of the temporal area, and (3) little or no pull on the upper part of the forehead and therefore with minimal hairline recession. The desired position of the eyebrows is carefully maintained during the 40 seconds required for the gluing (Fig. 6-2, *B*).

When there is considerable sagging of the lateral part of the eyebrow, a 3.0 nonabsorbable suture can be passed through the deep layer of the undermined temporal tissues at the eyebrow level. The stitch is then attached to the upper part of the temporal aponeurosis and tied after the gluing as additional support.

Closure

The incisions are closed with 4.0 Vicryl Rapide (Ethicon, Somerville, N.J.). No dressing is applied. It is important to instruct the patient and the nurses not to clean or rub the forehead for 24 hours to avoid ungluing the repositioned forehead. After 48 hours, a shampoo is allowed and can be repeated as frequently as desired.

Data Analysis and Evaluation

We performed 668 endoforehead procedures from November 1993 through June 2002. There were 653 females and 15 males. Of these 668 procedures, 664 were in association with a facelift and 64 were isolated endoforehead lifts. Most patients have been seen again for follow-up. Among the 452 patients seen after a minimum of 6 months following surgery, 140 patients were available for full evaluation.

Preoperatively and postoperatively, we measured the position of the eyebrows and muscle strength. The position of the eyebrows was calculated by noting the horizontal distance between the eyebrows and the vertical distance between the inner, median, and lateral lower part of the eyebrows to the inner canthus, pupil, and lateral canthus (Fig. 6-3). Muscle strength was evaluated by asking

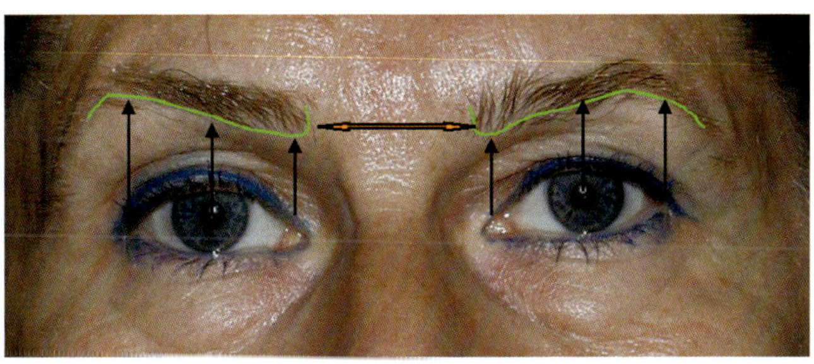

Figure 6-3 Distances are measured between the medial part of the eyebrows, the lateral and medial canthi to eyebrows, and the pupil to eyebrows.

the patient to frown and lift his or her eyebrows and was rated from 1 (weak) to 4 (very strong). We had estimated preoperatively from an aesthetic viewpoint the ideal displacement in terms of eyebrow elevation and lateral displacement. We compared these measurements with the early and late postoperative results.

The quality of eyebrow repositioning and muscle weakening—the two elements that were quantified—are given a score of 1 to 4 (1 = excellent, 2 = good, 3 = mediocre, 4 = poor). This rating is done by comparing the preoperative and postoperative measurements but also by clinical and photographic comparison of the preoperative and postoperative condition at a minimum of 6 months after the operation.

We have analyzed specifically:

1. The quality of the results in three groups of patients: Group A, 28 patients operated on during the first 6 months (November 1993 to May 1994); group B, 69 patients operated on during the next 18 months (May 1994 to November 1995); and group C, 43 patients operated on from January 1999 to July 1999
2. The incidence and nature of secondary procedures
3. The rate and evolution of complications

A simultaneous midface elevation after extensive subperiosteal dissection was performed in 18 patients. Fixation was made with heavy stitches passed from midface to the temporal fascia.

In two patients we used a biplanar approach to the forehead with a precapillary incision in cases of significant horizontal wrinkling associated with a high forehead.

Results

The evaluation consisted of (1) assessment of eyebrow position and morphologic results and (2) weakening of the frowning muscles. There was a striking difference between the first and second group, with a sharp increase in excellent results from 32% to 78% for eyebrow position and from 28% to 72% for muscle weakening. For the last group (1999) these figures increased slightly to 79% for eyebrow position and 81% for muscle weakening. One can say that the results in the last group represent only a minor improvement compared to the improvement seen between the first and second groups, and that the learning curve was short (Fig. 6-4).

Complications have not been significant. Two hematomas requiring aspiration were noted in the 668 endoforehead lifts. Ecchymoses were sometimes significant. Immediate postoperative pain requiring strong sedation was observed in 20% of the patients the first night. Of the 668 patients, 20% also complained of

A

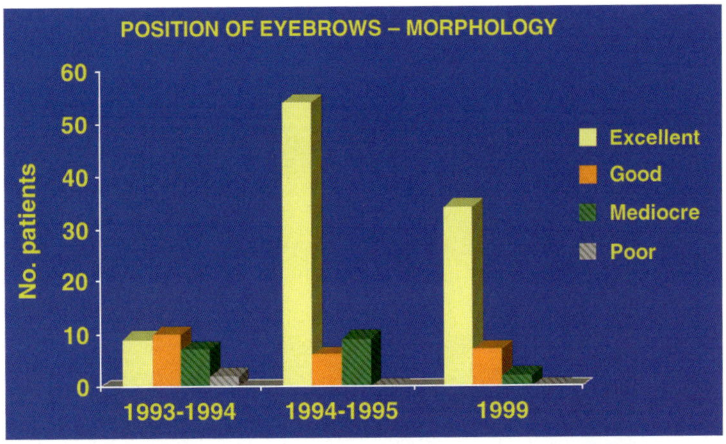

B

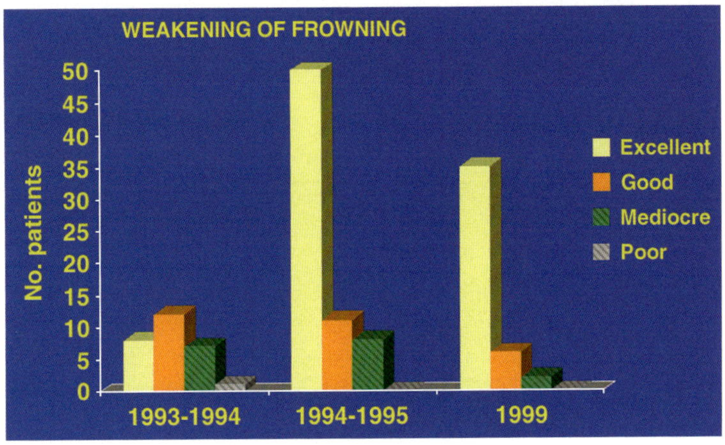

Figure 6-4 Comparison of the three groups evaluated. **A,** Position of eyebrows—morphology. **B,** Weakening of frowning.

unpleasant sensations of tightness or itching for a few weeks. In 3 of the 668 patients, scalp lesions due to scratching were observed. The skin of the eyelids is thin, and two accidental skin perforations occurred. They healed inconspicuously. Frontal facial palsy is the major complication that may be encountered with endoscopic—or for that matter, open—frontal lifts. During the first 3 years (1993 to 1996), we observed 5 palsies out of 206 patients. During the last 6 years (1996 to 2002), we observed only 3 cases of our 462 patients. All these frontal palsies were transient, and full recovery was obtained within 3 to 8 weeks.

The number of reoperations has also decreased with experience: in the first group, 6%; in the second group, 4%; and in the last group of 571 patients, only 3%. By reoperation we mean a re-elevation of the browlift, mainly because the first elevation of the brows was not sufficient and/or their new position was not maintained. These reoperations were not difficult, and the periosteum was easily elevated. There is occasionally some fibrous tissue at the corregator level, but dissection is still usually performed without difficulty.

Case Examples

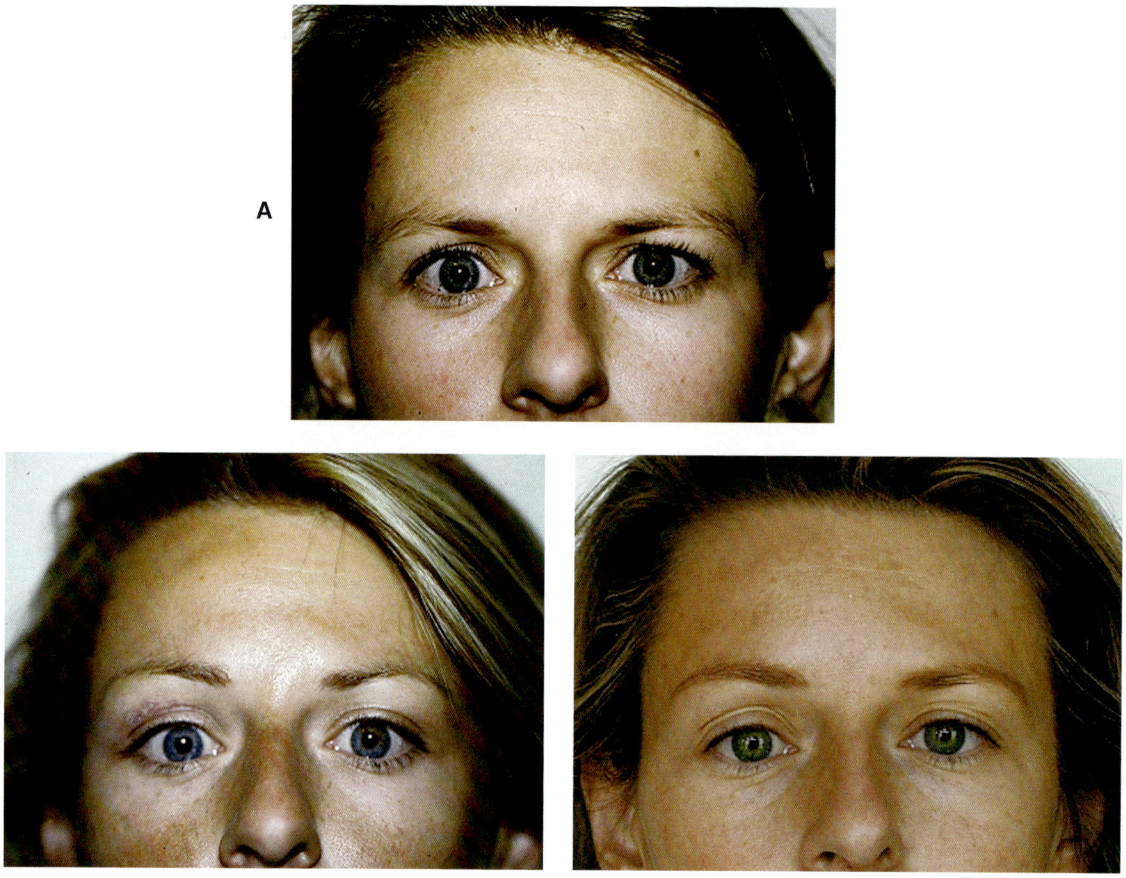

Before **(A)**, 6 months after **(B)**, and 5 years after **(C)** endoscopic forehead lift in a 31-year-old patient.

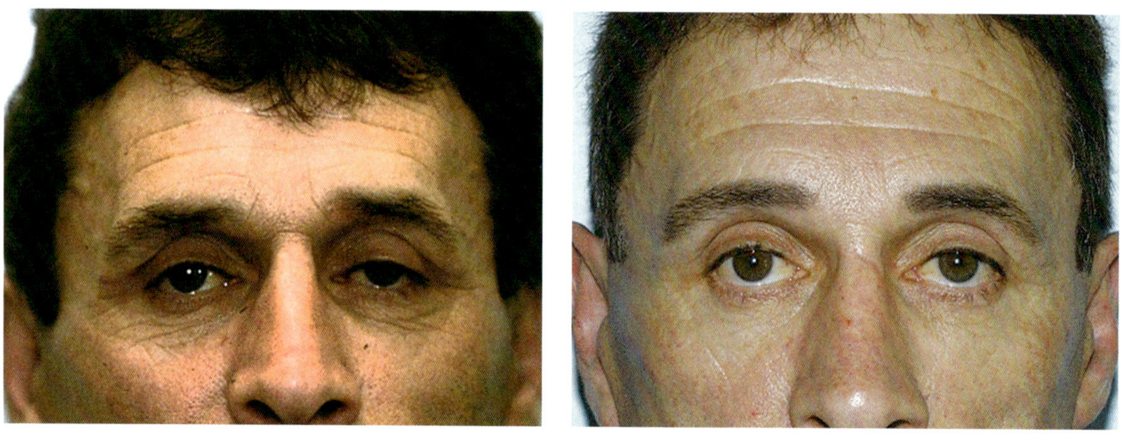

Before and 6 months after endoscopic forehead lift in a 53-year-old man.

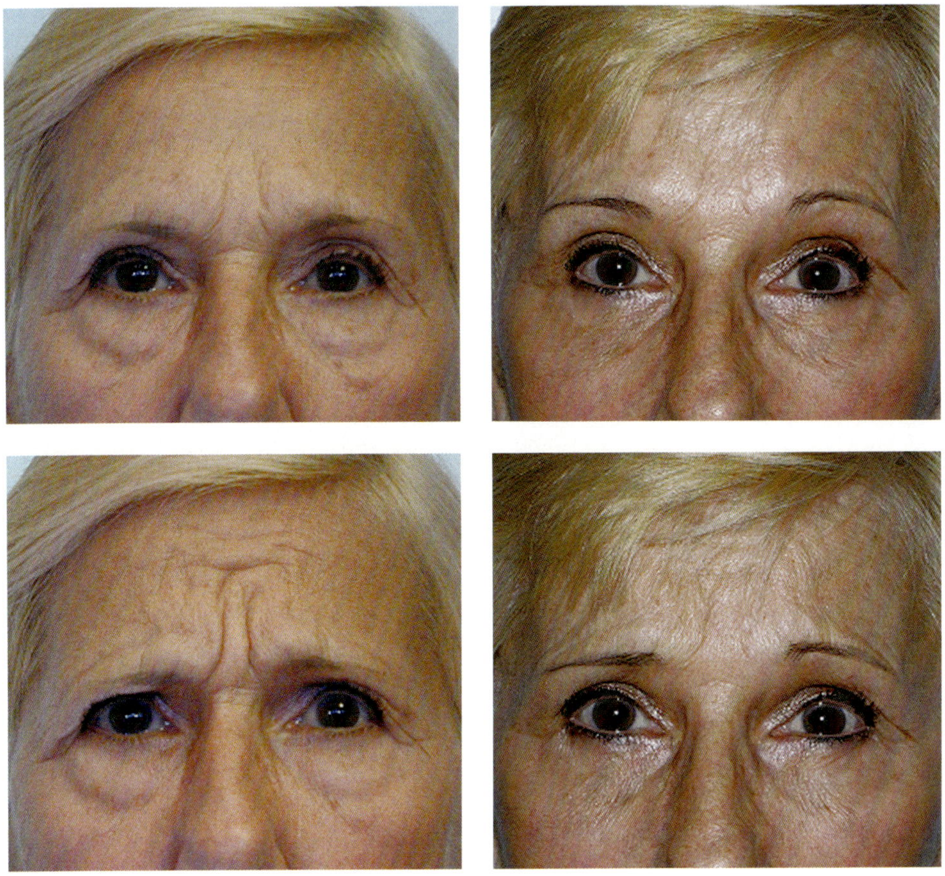

A 70-year-old woman, at rest and frowning before an endoscopic forehead lift and 6 months after the lift, at rest and frowning.

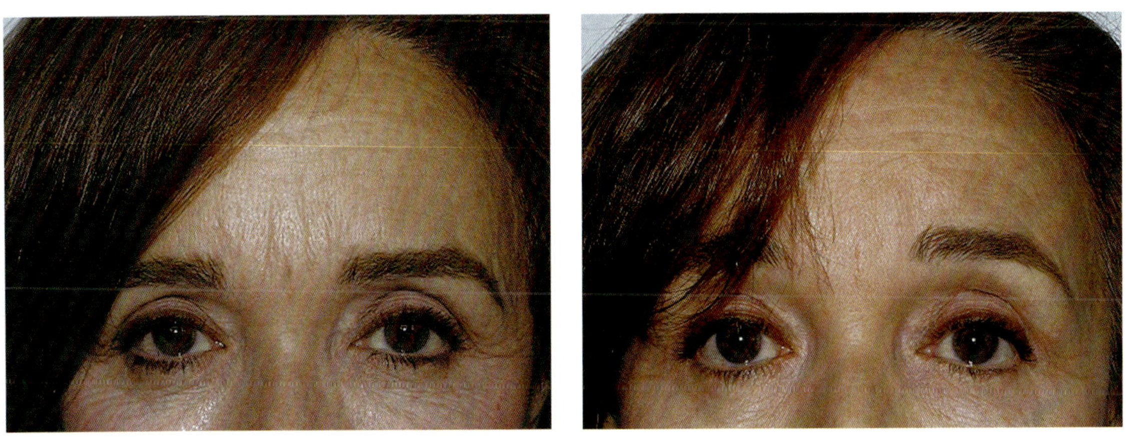

Before and 6 months after endoscopic forehead lift in a 60-year-old woman.

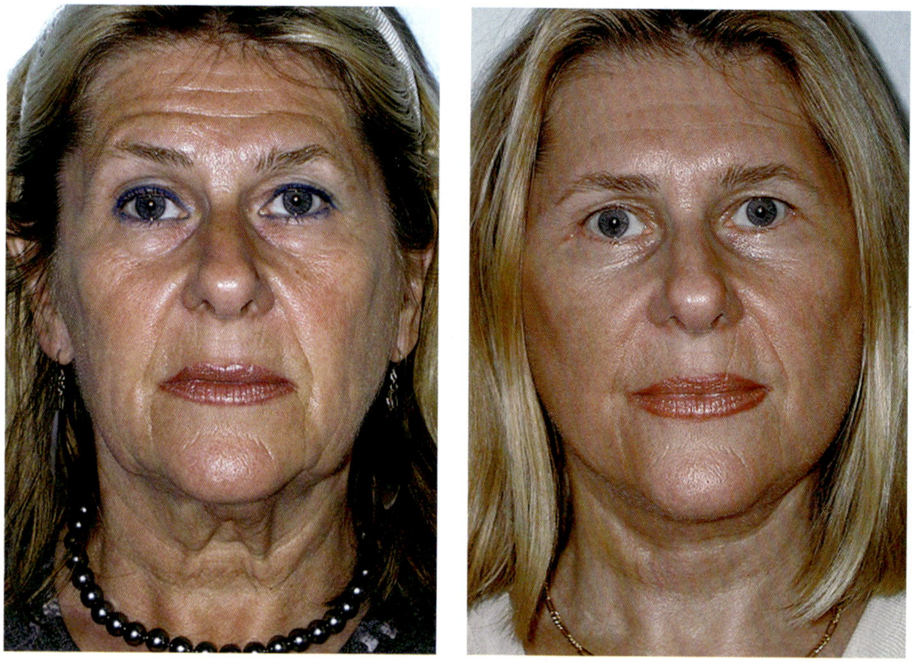

Association of a facelift and an endobrowlift gives better balance to the face and a more natural look. A 57-year-old woman before the operation and 20 days after the facelift and forehead lift.

Conclusion

The choice of an endoscopic approach versus a classic bicoronal approach remains an open issue since some surgeons (1) are not familiar with endoscopic techniques, (2) think that the coronal approach gives better results, or (3) think that an eyelid approach or a simple periosteal elevation without endoscopy is sufficient.

Our 7-year experience with the endoscopic forehead lift has been extremely positive. We have not done a single operation using the coronal approach for aesthetic purposes since 1993, when we began using the endoscopic technique. However, we routinely continue to use the coronal approach for craniofacial cases.

The endoscopic forehead lift is done quickly (in about 20 minutes) and provides a good and stable result for most patients, leaving practically no sequelae. Should reoperation become necessary, it can be done quickly and simply, in our experience.

The great advantage of fixation with fibrin glue, in addition to its simple application, is that the required displacement of the eyebrows can be made in different directions. Most patients benefit from transverse spreading of the glabellar area, which is associated with a moderate lateral elevation of the eyebrows. Traditional fixation with stitches and screws in an oblique direction limits these possibilities of adjustment and may easily lead to an excessive elevation of the brows.

We believe this endoscopic technique satisfies our patients' desires to look better and still keep a natural appearance (no signs of surgery). It must be stressed that in Europe the patients usually are concerned about not looking "operated on" and fear overcorrection, whereas in other parts of the world, patients look for a spectacular result. In terms of eyebrow elevation, it is obvious that when a significant upward displacement is planned, one can feel safer with fixation through screws or bony tunnels,[9-11] or even with skin staples, such as those used by Luis Vasconez,[12] rather than with the gluing technique.

REFERENCES

1. Vasconez LO, Core GB, Gumboa-Bobadilla M, Guzman G, Askren C, Yamamoto Y. Endoscopic techniques in coronal browlifting. Plast Reconstr Surg 94:788-793, 1994.
2. Isse NG. Endoscopic facial rejuvenation: Endoforehead, the functional lift. Case reports. Aesthetic Plast Surg 18:21-29, 1994.
3. Holle J, Freilinger G, Mandl H. The use of a fibrin glue adhesive system in plastic surgery. In Ely JF, ed. Transactions of the Seventh International Congress of Plastic and Reconstructive Surgery. Rio de Janeiro: Sociedad Brasileira Chirurgia Plastica, 1979.
4. Cruz NI, Debs N, Fiol RE. Evaluation of fibrin glue in rat sciatic nerve repairs. Plast Reconstr Surg 78:369-373, 1986.
5. Marchac D, Renier D. Fibrin glue in craniofacial surgery. J Craniofac Surg 1:32-34, 1990.
6. Marchac D, Sandor G. Face lifts and sprayed fibrin glue: An outcome analysis of 200 patients. Br J Plast Surg 47:306-309, 1994.
7. Marchac D, Pugash E, Gault D. The use of sprayed fibrin glue for face lifts. Eur J Plast Surg 10:139-143, 1987.
8. Marchac D, Ascherman J, Arnaud E. Fibrin glue fixation in forehead endoscopy: Evaluation of our experience with 206 cases. Plast Reconstr Surg 100:704-712, 1997.
9. Marchac D, Goni S. Endoscopic forehead lift. Acta Chir Belg 101:210-217, 2001.
10. Paul M. The evolution of the browlift in aesthetic plastic surgery. Plast Reconstr Surg 108: 1409-1423, 2001.
11. McKinney P, Sweis I. An accurate technique for fixation in endoscopic browlift: A 5-year follow-up. Plast Reconstr Surg 108:1808-1810, 2001.
12. Vasconez L, Anastasos J. Discussion of: "An accurate technique for fixation in endoscopic browlift: A 5-year follow-up." Plast Reconstr Surg 108:1811, 2001.

CHAPTER

7

Tissue Adhesive in Forehead Fixation With Endoscopic Forehead Lift

David A.F. Ellis, M.D., F.R.C.S.C.

Fibrin glues and sealants have been used for many years around the world. They recently have been introduced in the United States. Fibrin sealants are instrumental in three important wound-healing aspects:

1. Promote hemostasis
2. Effectively bind tissue
3. Support and aid wound healing

In the past decade there has been a desire to raise the eyebrows to make the eyes appear "bright eyed and bushy tailed" through a technique of endoscopic forehead lifting using fixation techniques to hold the eyebrows in their natural place. After several years and many surgical outcomes, this has resulted in multiple techniques in forehead fixation. None of the techniques actually fix the eyebrows at the level of the bony orbital ridge. The fibrin sealant does that. There is no concern about overcorrection or relapse.

Indications for Use

With a large surface area of undermining in the subperiosteal plane, fibrin glue is an ideal sealant with which to reattach the periosteum. Each eyebrow can be fixed in an exact position but different from the other when necessary. With 4 ml of mixture, both the central and lateral aspects of the eyebrow can be fixed. With suture techniques it is difficult to fix the lateral aspect of the eyebrow. With fibrin glue, however, this becomes technically easier and more predictable. The sealant has both adhesive properties and factors to aid healing. As the tensile strength of the adhesion is 22 psi, it is effective in the heavy brow skin.[1]

Preparation of Material

In Canada the mixture can be prepared in both slow-acting and fast-acting modes. The fast-acting glue formulation is used in forehead fixation. In the United States, only the fast-acting sealant is available. The 2 ml kit is used which makes 4 ml of sealant. In Canada only Tisseel (Baxter Corporation, Deerfield, Ill.) is available as a fibrin sealant. In the United States, both Tisseel and Hemaseel (Haemacure Corporation, Montreal, Quebec, Canada) are available as fibrin sealants, but essentially they are identical products. Tisseel comes with four bottles: two bottles have a black cap, and two bottles have a blue cap. The small black-capped bottle contains 2 ml of calcium chloride. The large black-capped bottle contains 2 ml of thrombin 500. (In Canada there is another silver-capped bottle that contains 2 ml of thrombin 4. This bottle is used for the slow-acting fibrin glue.) The small blue-capped bottle contains 2 ml of sterile bovine aprotinin solution at a concentration of 3000 kallikrein inhibitor units (KIU)/ml. The large blue-capped bottle contains 2 ml of Tisseel. This bottle contains factor XIII, fibrinogen, plasma fibronectin, and plasminogen.

In the reconstitution of the product the small blue-capped bottle is mixed into the large blue-capped bottle and placed in the Fibrinotherm warming device (Baxter Corporation), and the small black-capped bottle is mixed into the large black-capped bottle and placed in the Fibrinotherm warming device in the stirring socket. It remains there for 10 to 15 minutes. It is important not to let the Tisseel and aprotinin mixture froth. The stirrer on the Fibrinotherm warming device must be turned off if frothing occurs. With the new syringes supplied in the kit, 2 ml is drawn up from each bottle without inverting the bottles and each syringe is put in the Duploject Clip. Adding 1 ml of air above the solution will create a positive pressure so the solution can be easily removed. The company does not recommend this maneuver but I have found it to be very useful, and it does not alter the adhesive properties of the sealant. The 10 cm 20-gauge DuploTip is applied to the syringes on the Duploject Clip. The 10 cm 20-gauge DuploTip is a semirigid double-lumen catheter that carries each product separately down to the end where they meet and mix, causing the two surfaces to stick to one another.

The chemical reaction of fibrin glue mimics the pathway of the coagulation cascade without the red blood cells. In the black-capped bottle is 2 ml of calcium chloride and thrombin (500 IU/ml). In the blue-capped bottle is Tisseel with the aprotinin. When the contents of the two bottles are together at the end of the syringe, a tightly meshed polymer fibrin is formed that promotes hemostasis and tissue bonding and supports and aids normal wound healing. When the thrombin is mixed with the fibrinogen, a loose monomeric fibrin is formed. Under the influence of factor XIII and calcium chloride, the tightly meshed fibrin clot is formed. The normal degradation is blocked by aprotinin.[2] The clot with its adhesive properties remains until it becomes absorbed in about 10 to 14 days, at which time normal physiology takes over.

Timing in Use of Materials

The glue is applied after full dissection, release of the scalp, and adequate wrinkle control. Immediately after the application of the sealant, the incisions are closed.

Application of Tissue Glues

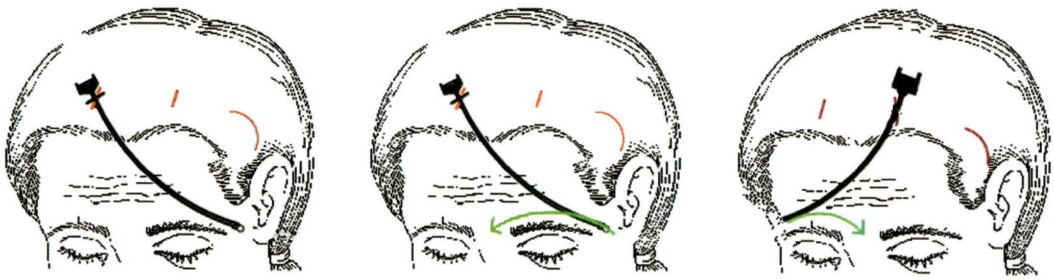

The double cannula is inserted in the left or right central incisional openings with the tip below and lateral to the lateral part of the eyebrow. The sealant is squeezed out, fixing the lateral part of the eyebrow, and the tip is then moved medially below the eyebrow to the glabella area.

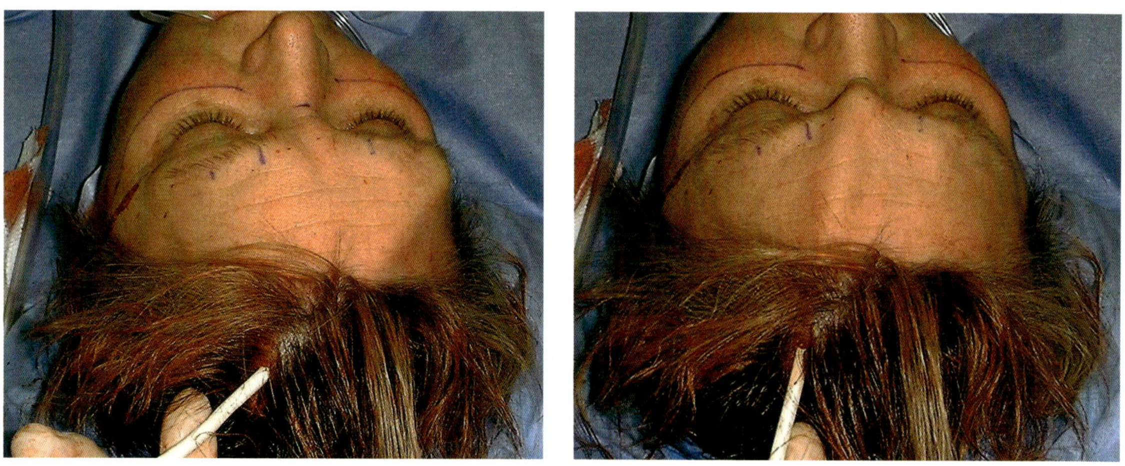

Note the depth of the cannula. It is below the brow and starts lateral to the brow and ends in the glabella area.

Preparation of Wound

A well-executed forehead lift requires four elements:

1. Proper selection of patients
2. Adequate dissection and release of the scalp from the underlying structures
3. Performance of adequate wrinkle control
4. Fixation

Before the application of the glue, full dissection and subperiosteal release of the scalp from the bony margins must be completed. Anteriorly this dissection must be carried inferior to the bony orbital margin, avoiding damage to the supraorbital nerve. The dissection is then taken through the periosteum into the subcutaneous pocket, which contains fat below the level of the eyebrow. Posteriorly the dissection is taken back to the nuchal line. Wrinkle control is achieved after full release in the subperiosteal plane. If there is a lot of lateral brow ptosis, the lateral orbicularis fibers can be transected multiple times without damage to the superficial skin. This is done with electrocautery and a long 4-inch curved Colorado needle. Medial wrinkle control for the depressors and frown lines is done in two steps: The first is electrocautery of the nerve to the corrugator muscle as it enters the superior aspect of the lateral part of the corrugator muscle. This is consistently located 1 to 1.6 cm above the lower border of the eyebrow 1 cm lateral to the supraorbital notch.[3] This effectively removes the horizontal component of frowning. The second is to weaken the depressor function of frowning. Electrocautery dicing of the superior medial aspect of the orbicularis oculi muscle and procerus muscle is done without damage to the superficial skin. For the 18 months leading up to December 1997, I recalled 9 of 27 patients after a minimum of 2 years after cutting the nerve to the corrugator muscle to evaluate this muscle-weakening technique. Five cases were performed endoscopically, three were performed via a transbrow approach, and one was performed through a pretrichial incision. The happiness factor averaged 4.6 out of 5 with a range from 4 to 5. The horizontal component of frowning averaged 0.9 out of 5 with a range of 0 to 3. The depressor component of frowning averaged 3 out of 5 with a range of 2 to 5. This indicates that cutting the nerve to the corrugator muscle is a more permanent solution than just dicing the muscle and significantly alters the horizontal component of frowning.

Surgical Technique

Prior to the surgery, the surgeon and the patient will have discussed the exact desired position of each eyebrow. Some like their eyebrows higher laterally, but most wanted a symmetrical elevation of the brow. For asymmetrical elevation the glue is an ideal way of creating more balance and precision in positioning the eyebrows.

The brows should be manipulated so that the exact position where they will be glued can be visualized. A 10 cm stiff but flexible double cannula is attached to the end of the two-syringe holder. One side is glued at a time. The left side is glued by putting the double cannula in through the right or left central incision. The cannula tip is placed laterally below the lateral aspect of the eyebrow. Initially 1 ml of sealant is squeezed out and manually spread superiorly to fix the lateral eyebrow and the skin above it to the deep temporal fascia. This can be facilitated by moving the cannula tip superiorly. It is important to fix the lateral aspect of the brow. To fix the medial part of the brow, the cannula tip is then slid medially, running the tip below the brow to the glabella area. The hand can be used to spread the sealant superiorly. I use 1 ml in this maneuver. The same procedure is used on the other side. On each side 2 ml of sealant is used. After the forehead is sealed, pressure is maintained for 3 minutes while stapling or suturing the incisions. A 3-inch elastic bandage is wrapped around the forehead as a dressing.

I evaluated the 2-year postendoscopic forehead cases treated with sealant fixation only in the years 1998 and 1999. There were 68 cases treated, and in a 2-year period 15 of these patients were recalled. All 15 patients were seen a minimum of 2 years after surgery. No patient had inadequate brow elevation, and none had returned to their preoperative status. There was no need for overcorrection, and the happiness factor was 14 out of 15 patients.

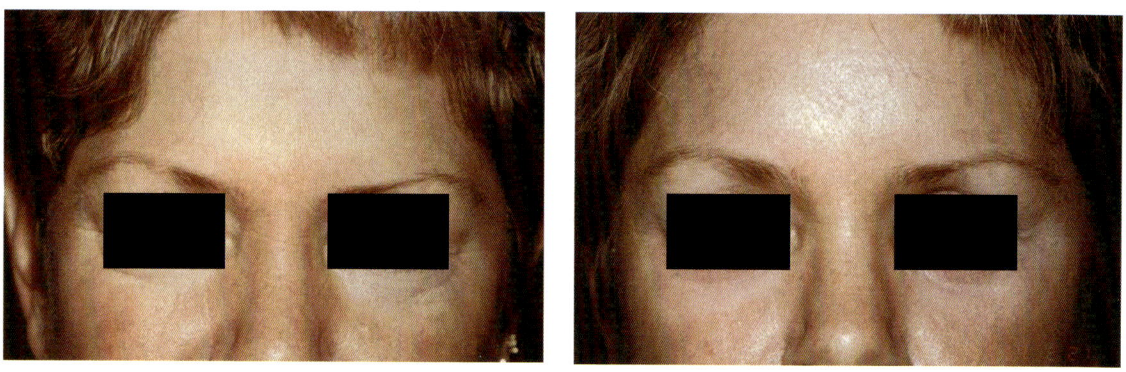

Endoscopic forehead lift was performed using Tisseel fixation to permit more upper eyelid visualization. Note the heavy brow skin.

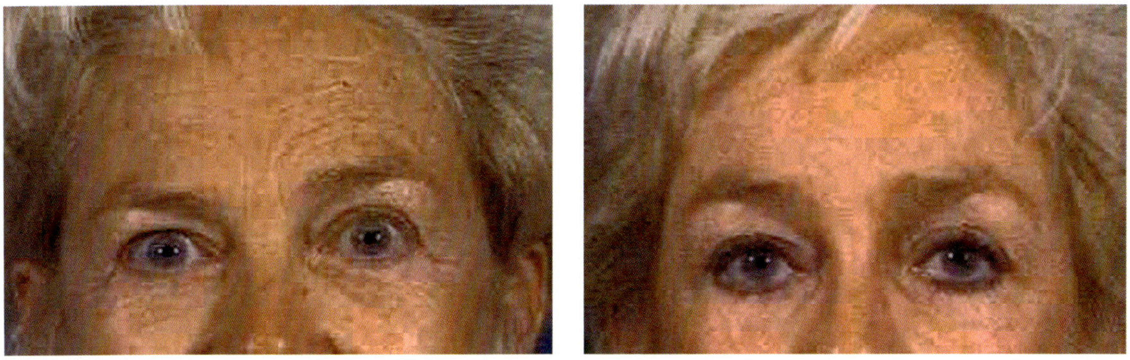

Asymmetric eyebrows were corrected with endoscopic forehead lift using Tisseel fixation. Full-face CO_2 laser was also performed.

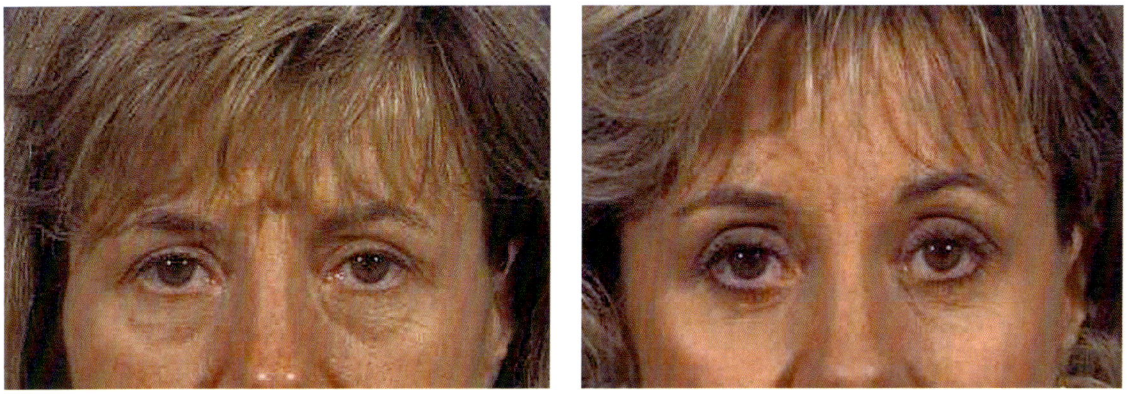

Endoscopic forehead lift using Tisseel fixation on the patient who wanted larger eyes.

Problems, Pitfalls, and Potential Complications

When the fast-acting sealant is used, the exact position of each eyebrow must be visualized and put into place before the addition of the glue. If the eyebrows are too asymmetrical or too low, then it is a simple technique of releasing the adhesion and regluing the brows in the desired position. Time will be wasted, however, as it may take 15 minutes to reconstitute another preparation.

The glue will not work if it is incorrectly prepared. In most hospital or private surgical facilities, however, nurses have been well trained to avoid this error.

Summary

1. Perform all the necessary dissection before using the sealant.
2. Plan exactly where you want the brows before applying the sealant.
3. Apply the sealant consistently in the manner described above.
4. Apply pressure for 3 minutes.

Conclusion

In facial cosmetic surgery, I believe the best way to fix the position of the eyebrows is with the use of a fibrin sealant. Each brow can be fixed exactly at the supraorbital rim where the patient desires his or her eyebrows. Also, fibrin sealant is a great benefit in facelift procedures, as it speeds healing and decreases the amount of swelling, thus shortening the "down time." In rhinoplasty, it is ideal for gluing cartilaginous tip grafts, as gluing is faster and more precise than suturing, and there is no chance for a piece of cartilage to become displaced. Midface and malar implants have been fixed with fibrin glue for the past decade without a single problem. In cases in which a nasal dorsal implant needs to be centered, the surgeon can remove the implant, center the pocket, and use fibrin sealant to keep the implant centered all in one operation.

In facial reconstructive surgery, the fibrin sealant can be used effectively in large and small flaps to help control small-vessel oozing and speed healing. It is worthwhile with skin grafts, as no bolsters are needed. The fibrin sealant not only aids and supports healing of the skin graft but also helps to stick the graft firmly to its base. It can also be used in facial nerve grafts.

References

1. Redl H, Schlag G. Properties of different tissue sealants with special emphasis on fibrinogen-based preparations. Fibrin Sealant in Operative Medicine, vol. 1. Berlin: Springer-Verlag, 1995, pp 27-38.
2. Tisseel Kit VH package insert.
3. Ellis DAF, Bakala CB. Anatomy of the motor innervation of the corrugator supercilii muscle: Clinical significance and development of a new surgical technique for frowning. J Otolaryngol 27:222-227, 1998.

CHAPTER

8

USE OF FIBRIN SEALANT IN SHORT SCAR FACELIFT

Alan Matarasso, M.D. ▪ Samieh S. Rizk, M.D.

As this textbook illustrates, fibrin sealants have been used in surgical procedures for decades. First applied in intracranial surgery in 1915,[1] they have also been used in otolaryngologic surgery for sealing cerebrospinal fluid leaks, thoracic surgery for primary repair of thoracic duct leaks and esophageal anastomoses,[2] general surgery for colostomy closure and splenic repair, orthopedic surgery for tendon repairs,[3] and plastic surgery for skin grafts,[4] rhytidectomy,[5] blepharoplasty,[6] and endoscopic forehead lift.[7] Fibrin glue's success in limiting hematoma and seroma formation, while abolishing the need for drains in rhytidectomy, has brought this agent to the attention of aesthetic surgeons. The potential for a more rapid recovery postoperatively has further popularized it.

This chapter focuses on the role of fibrin sealant, or "tissue glue," in short scar facelift. We began using fibrin sealants over a decade ago, but until recently they were not standard in our practice. With regard to the use of the short scar incision, it has always been our practice in younger patients to perform an "upper" facelift where the incision begins on the temporal hairline, with or without a sideburn cut, and ends in the postlobule sulcus. It is only more recently, however, that we have applied the short transauricular rhytidectomy, without any hair-bearing incisions, in all patients regardless of degree of deformity, age, gender, or prior surgical history.

Although the debate continues to rage as to the optimal facelift procedure, many would agree that the ideal procedure would be one that produces the shortest scar with the least morbidity and the best result. Patients' desire for less invasive procedures with faster recoveries has served as an ongoing impetus for innovations in aesthetic surgery. Our primary motivation for incorporating the tissue sealant into the short scar facelift technique was to improve the coaptation of the dissected surfaces and to enhance flap redraping.[8-10] With this limited incision approach, there are three key principles. First, we continue to advocate wide skin undermining as well as redraping and repositioning of the superficial musculoaponeurotic system (SMAS)-platysma layer. Second, laxity of the anterior neck is often addressed with a midline anterior platysma muscle resection and concomitant submentalplasty procedure with or without deep fat excision. Finally, an alteration in flap redraping with a more vertical vector than the traditional facelift approach, while adjusting the flap for dog ears, and closure of the dead space with fibrin tissue sealant are key factors. In addition to these principles, electrocautery is widely incorporated for subcutaneous tissue contouring and hemostasis. The addition of fibrin sealant (Tisseel, Baxter Corporation, Deerfield, Ill.) to facelift surgery in our practice has eliminated the use of drains in all cases. As has been reported, fibrin sealants have reduced bruising, edema, pain, hematoma, and seroma formation, enabling a more rapid recovery.

The evolution of the facelift incision into the short scar and the adjunctive use of fibrin sealant has advantages such as diminished ecchymosis and edema, with a subsequent faster recovery. Additionally, the fibrin component allows it to seal the large raw surface created during rhytidectomy and to stop oozing from smaller vessels, thus minimizing seromas, hematomas, bruising, and edema. Perhaps the most alluring advantage for patients who undergo the short scar facelift is the freedom it allows women to style and wear their hair up without altering their hairline position and men to obtain short haircuts without concern that a hairline scar or distortion might be exposed.

Fibrin Sealant Basic Physiology

Fibrin sealant is a physiologic, nontoxic hemostatic agent that is partially derived from human plasma. The sealant components of human fibrinogen, human thrombin, and bovine aprotinin stimulate the natural process of healing by simulating clot formation at the final phase of coagulation.[3] Given its derivation, however, the fear of viral transmission initially limited its use. Although viral transmission remains theoretically possible, several measures have been taken to virtually eliminate this possibility. Careful selection of plasma donors who are tested for viral serology serially over time, followed by a two-step vapor heating process of screened samples, helps maintain an excellent safety profile.[11] Fibrin sealant has been used in more than eight million surgical procedures since it was first marketed in 1983, and to date there have been no confirmed cases of HIV or hepatitis A, B, or C acquired from its use.[11,12] Introduction of the spray applicator to facilitate mixing of the product and the atomizer to evenly distribute the sealant has also contributed to the acceptance of this product.

Indications for Use

Fibrin sealant firmly adheres to connective tissue and has elastic properties that enable it to contour over pulsating areas. It is ideal for use over small areas of oozing but is not indicated for arterial bleeding. Fibrin sealant is indicated for controlling oozing on large raw surfaces.[12] It has not been associated with any caustic tissue damage when it is applied locally and is completely absorbed within 1 to 2 weeks.[13] Early forms of fibrin sealant had higher sodium content that rendered the clots formed transparent, and more brittle. The low sodium content of newer formulations enables the thrombin to convert the fibrinogen to fibrin on the tissue surface. This creates a fibrin matrix with structured strands that are more effectively cross-linked by factor XIIIa, forming a stronger visible clot.[13] Once the clot is formed, the bovine aprotinin component, an antifibrinolytic agent, reduces the rate of clot lysis by endogenous plasmin.[14] By sealing the raw surfaces of capillaries, postoperative bleeding, edema, pain, and the potential for hematoma formation are minimized.

Timing and Application of Sealant

The spray application device allows maximal mixing and application of a thin layer of sealant. A thinner, less dense layer of fibrin is recommended to provide a more physiologic approximation of tissue and thus facilitate wound healing.[7] A single 2 ml package applied with the dual-injection system can cover a surface area of approximately 200 cm^2. The cost is partially offset by the savings from omitted drainage tubes and decreased recovery time.[15] Once it is evenly sprayed, the skin flap is held in position for 3 minutes until set into position. The 45-minute preparation time can easily be performed during surgery by ancillary nursing staff, but the sealant must be maintained at 37° C after preparation. If the product cools, it becomes more viscous, and effective application is compromised.[3]

It is possible to extract the patient's own fibrinogen preoperatively to prepare autologous fibrin sealant. Indeed, our first experience with tissue sealants over a decade ago was with these products. One commercially available kit enables the physician to extract 4 ml of fibrin sealant from 120 ml of the patient's plasma[16]; however, this process is time consuming and requires more perioperative planning. Other available hemostatic agents include the following: autologous platelet-rich plasma combined with bovine thrombin and calcium chloride (platelet gel), autologous platelet-poor plasma rich in fibrinogen mixed with thrombin and calcium chloride in a 10:1 concentration (fibrin glue), and exogenous human or bovine thrombin spray.[16,17] Autologous platelet gel and fibrin glue require preparation in an autotransfusion machine utilizing automated centrifugation and are less effective hemostatic agents than commercially available preparations.[16]

Preparation of Material

Tisseel VH fibrin sealant comes prepackaged with four vials in each kit: a sealer protein concentrate (human), a fibrinolysis inhibitor solution (bovine), thrombin (human), and a calcium chloride solution (Fig. 8-1, *A*). Thrombin is

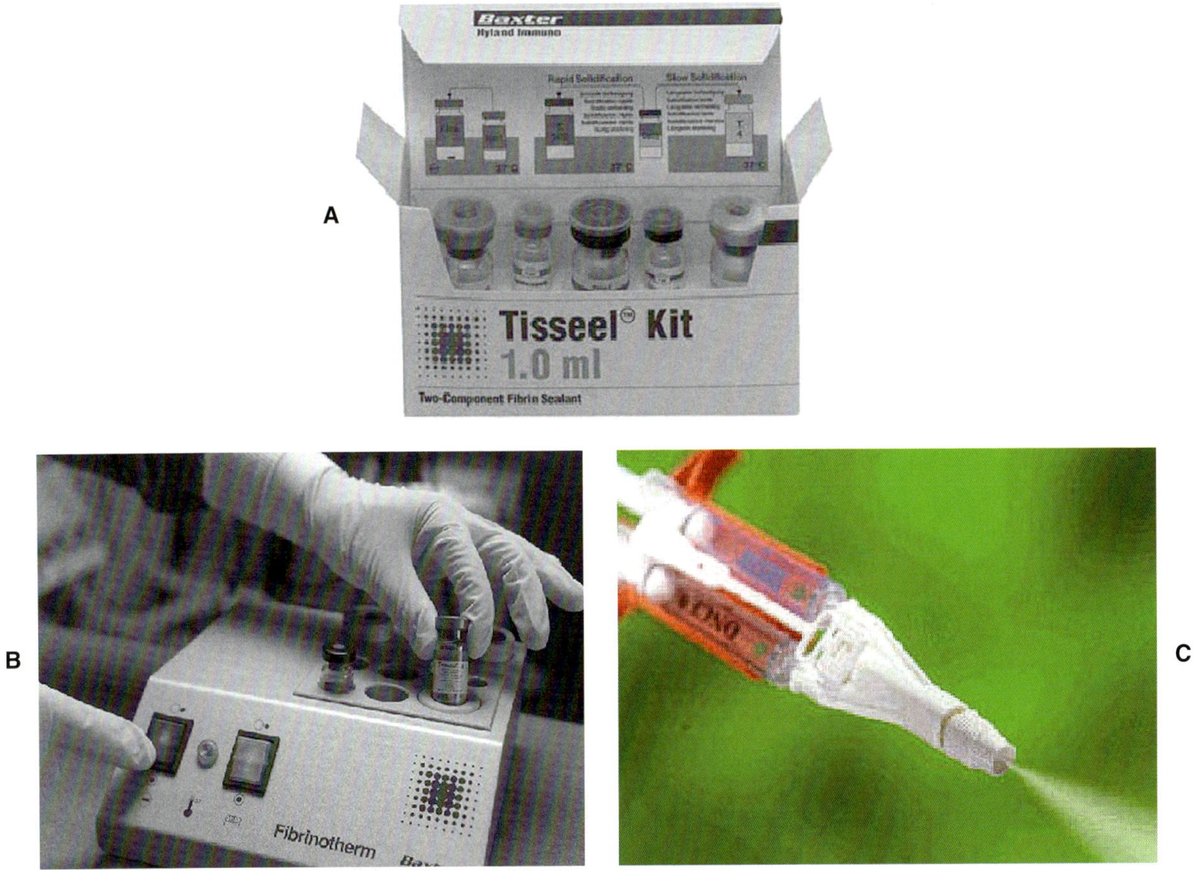

Figure 8-1 **A,** Fibrin sealant kit. **B,** Heating device for sealant. **C,** Dual-projection delivery aerosolizing syringes.

an enzyme that converts fibrinogen into fibrin, which is stabilized by the fibrinolysis-inhibitor enzyme. Preparation of the glue involves heating the sealer protein and fibrinolysis inhibitor for 10 minutes and then mixing them together to make the sealer protein solution. The device for heating and mixing these two substances is easy to use and has labels indicating where to place the various ingredients (Fig. 8-1, *B*). The thrombin and calcium chloride solution are then combined to form the thrombin solution. The sealer protein solution and the thrombin solution are then placed in separate syringes in the dual-injection device. The dual-injection device is then connected to the pressurized nitrogen gas tank, which aerosolizes the glue into a fine mist (Fig. 8-1, *C*). These two components are then sprayed together in equal amounts and mixed in the recipient tissue evenly on the flap and raw surfaces, where they polymerize to form the fibrin clot. The aerosolizing process prevents clumping for an even distribution of the glue into the recipient flap. A 2 ml kit is used for each facelift (0.75 ml per side and 0.50 for the submental wound). A 5 ml kit is also available.

Surgical Technique

The short scar facelift technique is a result of a continuous evolution from the traditional "open" facelift incision (Fig. 8-2, *A*), into the "modified" open technique (Fig. 8-2, *B*), and finally into the short scar facelift or the 5-STAR (short transauricular rhytidectomy) approach (Fig. 8-2, C). All of the patients who have had this short scar facelift also had concomitant suction-assisted lipoplasty (SAL) as indicated, and most (66%) underwent a submentalplasty. The short scar approach provides a shorter, more appealing, and well-hidden scar, essentially no hair abnormalities, potentially shorter operative time, and greater patient acceptance at the expense of a slightly narrower operative field with limited access to the orbicularis oculi muscle and temporalis muscle.

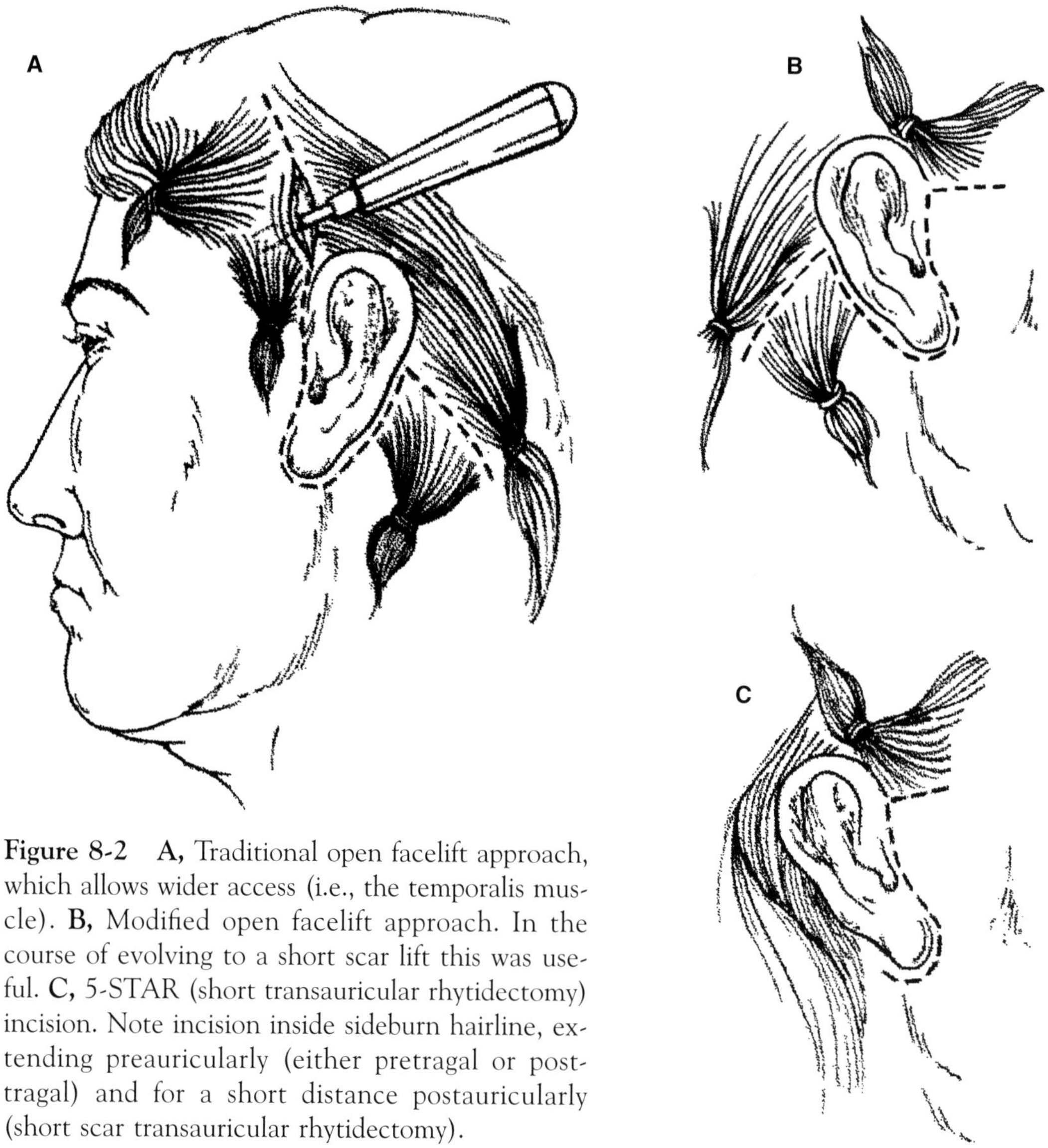

Figure 8-2 **A,** Traditional open facelift approach, which allows wider access (i.e., the temporalis muscle). **B,** Modified open facelift approach. In the course of evolving to a short scar lift this was useful. **C,** 5-STAR (short transauricular rhytidectomy) incision. Note incision inside sideburn hairline, extending preauricularly (either pretragal or posttragal) and for a short distance postauricularly (short scar transauricular rhytidectomy).

Incision Placement

The short scar incision begins in the horizontal aspect of the sideburn, extends to the preauricular region (either pretragal or post-tragal), curves around the ear lobe posteriorly up to the postauricular notch, ending 2 to 3 cm from the lobule. It spares incisions in the temporal, most of the postauricular sulcus, and the mastoid areas (see Fig. 8-2, C).

Preoperative Preparation

Sequential pneumatic compression devices are applied in all patients. Intravenous sedation is administered by the anesthesiologist, and local anesthesia (100 ml of normal saline, 100 ml of 1% lidocaine, and 1 ml of epinephrine) is injected by the surgeon. The patient is then prepared and draped, and povidone iodine (Betadine)–soaked cotton plugs are placed in the ear canals. Broad-spectrum systemic antibiotics are given.

Technique

The operation begins with liposuction of the neck with a 2.4 mm Mercedes cannula. Liposuction of any other facial sites is done with a 1.8 mm Mercedes cannula as indicated. Any necessary fat grafting or repositioning follows. The short scar facelift requires additional midline platysma work, accounting for the higher rate of submentalplasty than is done with the traditional facelift (66% vs. 10.6%) in our series. Through a submental incision the midline platysma is isolated, and a wide-strip wedge platysma excision is performed to shorten redundant platysma muscle. When submuscular fat excision is indicated, the exposed fat deep to the platysma muscle is excised under direct vision. The medial borders of the platysma muscle are then identified, and back-cut incisions are done in the muscle at the level of the hyoid bone. The medial borders of the platysma are then sutured in the midline with a nonabsorbable suture. This suturing begins inferiorly and runs continuously to the chin and is reinforced with a second layer of interrupted sutures. This medial vector pull on the platysma is important for defining the cervicomental angle and for the redraping of excess skin into the submental hollow that occurs with the short scar facelift. It is not necessary or desirable to have excess lateral vector pull on the platysma. During the evolution of the technique an ellipse of excess submental skin occasionally was removed at the submentalplasty incision. Later we used subcutaneous quilting sutures to tack the flap down, and we also used a drain through the submental incision. With the introduction of the tissue glue, these maneuvers became superfluous. The midline neck is opened at the beginning of surgery, and it is closed after all other incisions have been closed to allow observation for final hemostasis.

We have found that "fatty necks," after being aggressively defatted, often have a surprising degree of tissue elasticity and retraction, allowing less skin excision than would be expected. In contrast, thin necks in older patients with "chicken skin" lack elasticity, and have poor collagen structure in addition to the diminished number of pilosebaceous units. Consequently, no amount of excessive pulling or tightening will ultimately overcome these characteristics. Indeed, attempting to compensate in these situations by excessive pulling via any surgical approach is a futile exercise that does not benefit poor quality skin.

The face and neck skin is undermined widely beyond the sternocleidomastoid muscle and then across the cheek and along the jowl, freeing any retaining ligaments. The SMAS in the face is identified and addressed with either an SMAS resection, SMAS plication, or anterior imbrication. Final hemostasis and aggressive subcutaneous tissue contouring are performed with a ball tip electrocautery. Next, the skin flaps on one side are grasped at the level of the helix with an allis clamp and posteriorly with a skin hook. The flaps are then redraped obliquely (allis) and vertically (skin hook), so that the mandible no longer represents a "border" to the advancement of the neck skin (Fig. 8-3, *A*). This is done while adjusting the flap position to minimize bunching at the proximal (anterior end of the sideburn) and distal (posterior lobule) incisions.

After the SMAS is tightened and the skin flaps are rotated, positioned, trimmed, and tacked, the tissue glue is sprayed in an even, thin layer (0.75 ml per side) on the undersurface of the flap and on the raw dissected surfaces through the sideburn, preauricular, and postlobule incisions (Fig. 8-3, *B*). The fibrin sealant is sprayed in 60 seconds or less, and then external gentle pressure must be applied to the flaps with moist gauze for 3 minutes (Fig. 8-3, *C*) for a total time of 4 minutes. During this period the preauricular and transverse sideburn incisions are closed with 4.0 and 5.0 nylon running sutures, and the postlobule skin requires "walking out" toward the distal part of the incision as it is closed with staples. The addition of the tissue glue provides a significant draping advantage in the neck and postauricular region. At the completion of one side, the patient is turned and the other side is operated on. After repeating the process, we return our attention to the submental wound. The submental incision is again inspected, final hemostasis is obtained, and the remaining sealant is sprayed as described above. Approximately 1.5 ml of the sealant is used for both sides of the face (0.75 ml per side), and the remainder 0.5 ml is used in the submental pocket. A dressing consisting of three rows of open 4 × 8 gauze pads is applied and secured with a surgical net dressing.

Postoperative instructions include the following:

1. Vigorous pulmonary care, early ambulation, and supplemental oxygen
2. Analgesics, antiemetics, antihypertensives as indicated, and homeopathic medications
3. Limited activity; no bending or straining
4. Cold compresses
5. Routine hair care and grooming but no scrubbing of the face

A
B
C

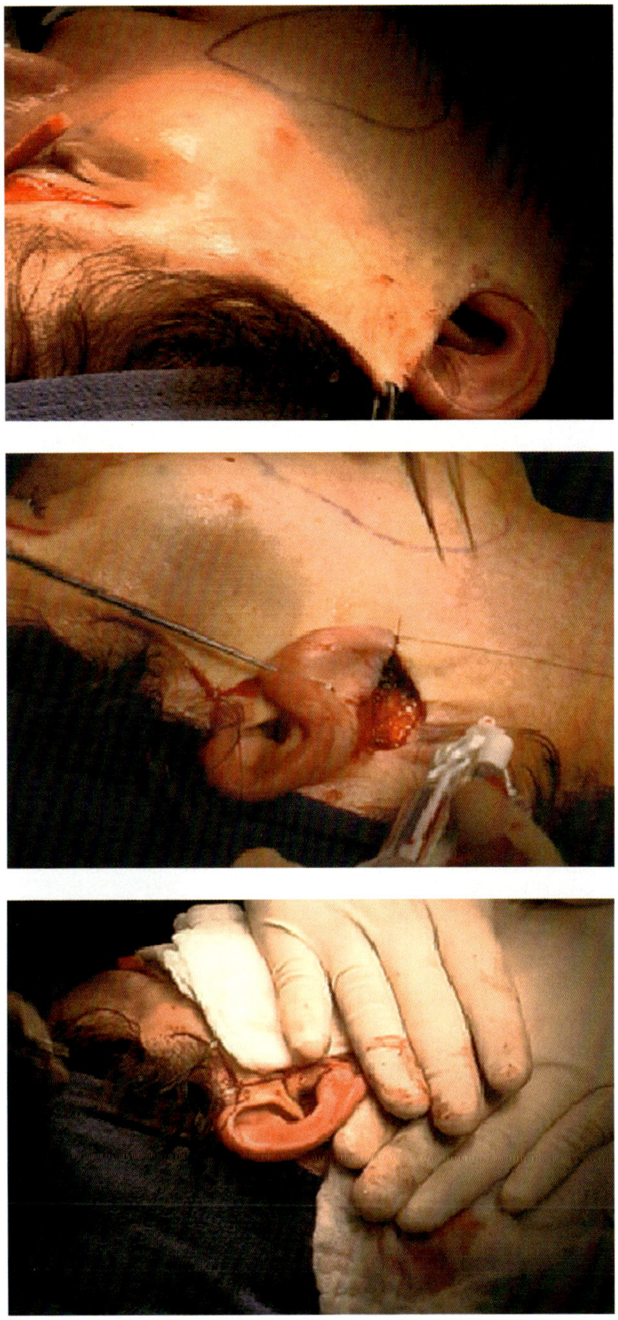

Figure 8-3 **A,** Flap redraping in an oblique and vertical vector prior to sealant application. Note the blue circle depicting the area of the jowl that was liposuctioned. **B,** Intraoperative fibrin sealant application with dual-injection device prior to closing. Key sutures at the helical rim and tragus. The preauricular suture begins at the lobule and is then used in a running fashion up to the helical rim. Note the redundant postauricular skin that redrapes and flattens. This is aided by the fibrin sealant and "walking out" the excess tissue while closing with staples. **C,** Fibrin sealant is applied within 1 minute and manual pressure for 3 minutes after application. During this time, wounds are closed.

Case Examples

The following are cases randomly selected from our series of 427 patients, illustrating the use of fibrin sealant in short scar facelift.

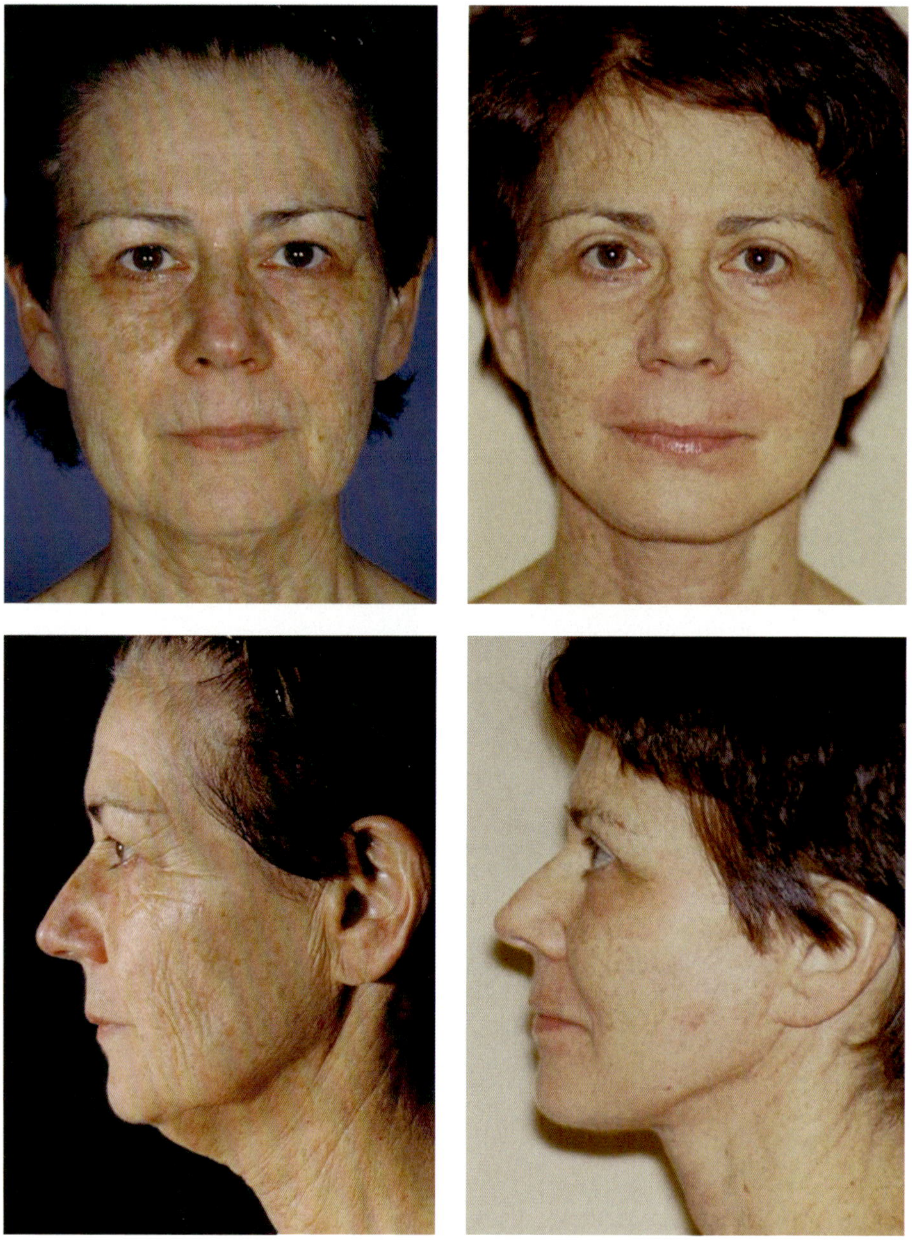

This is a 60-year-old woman who underwent short scar facelift, submentalplasty, upper and lower blepharoplasty, and periocular and perioral erbium laser skin resurfacing. Early postoperative views: Note the improvement in neck contour with the short scar facelift.

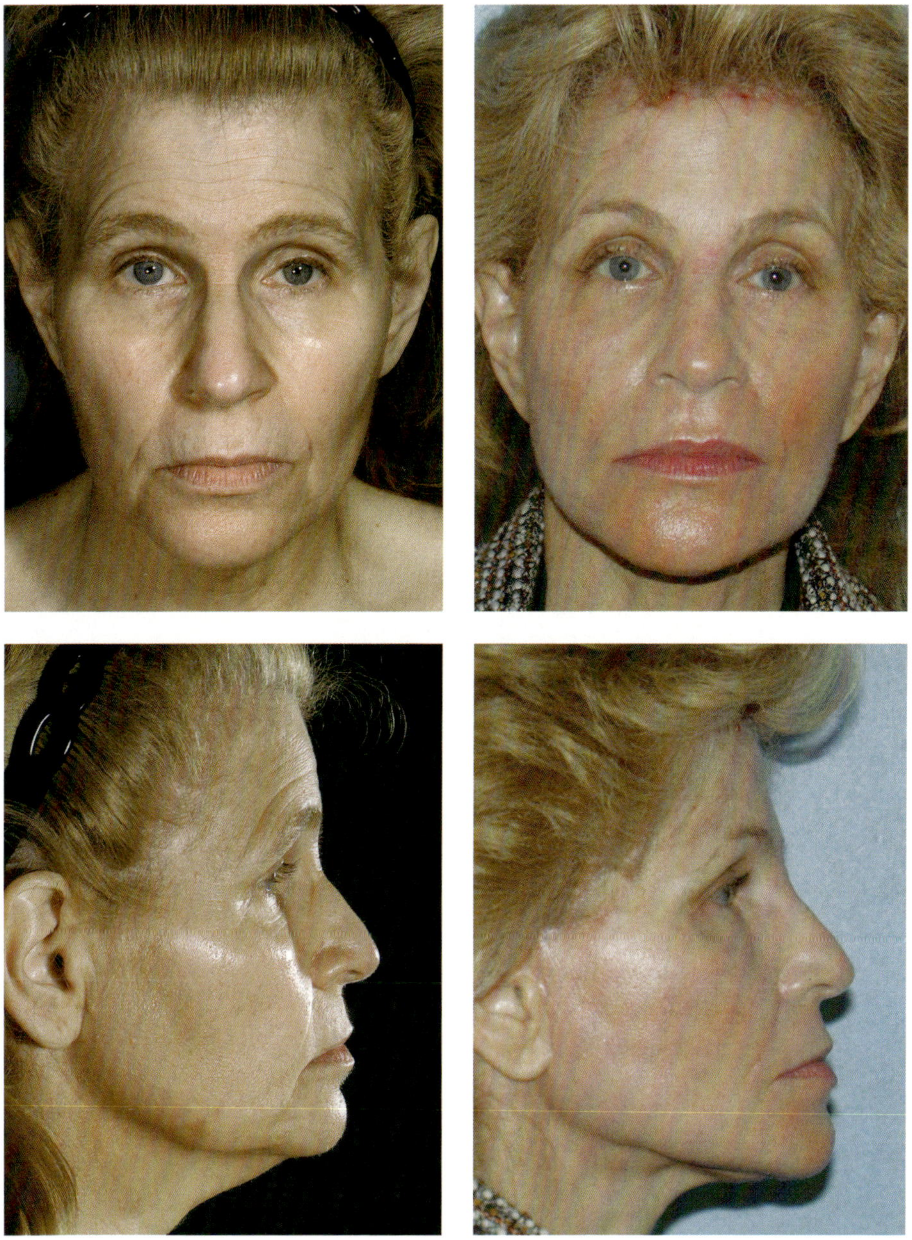

This is a 58-year-old woman who underwent a short scar facelift, submentalplasty, anterior browlift, and perioral erbium laser skin resurfacing. Postoperative views shown at 3 months.

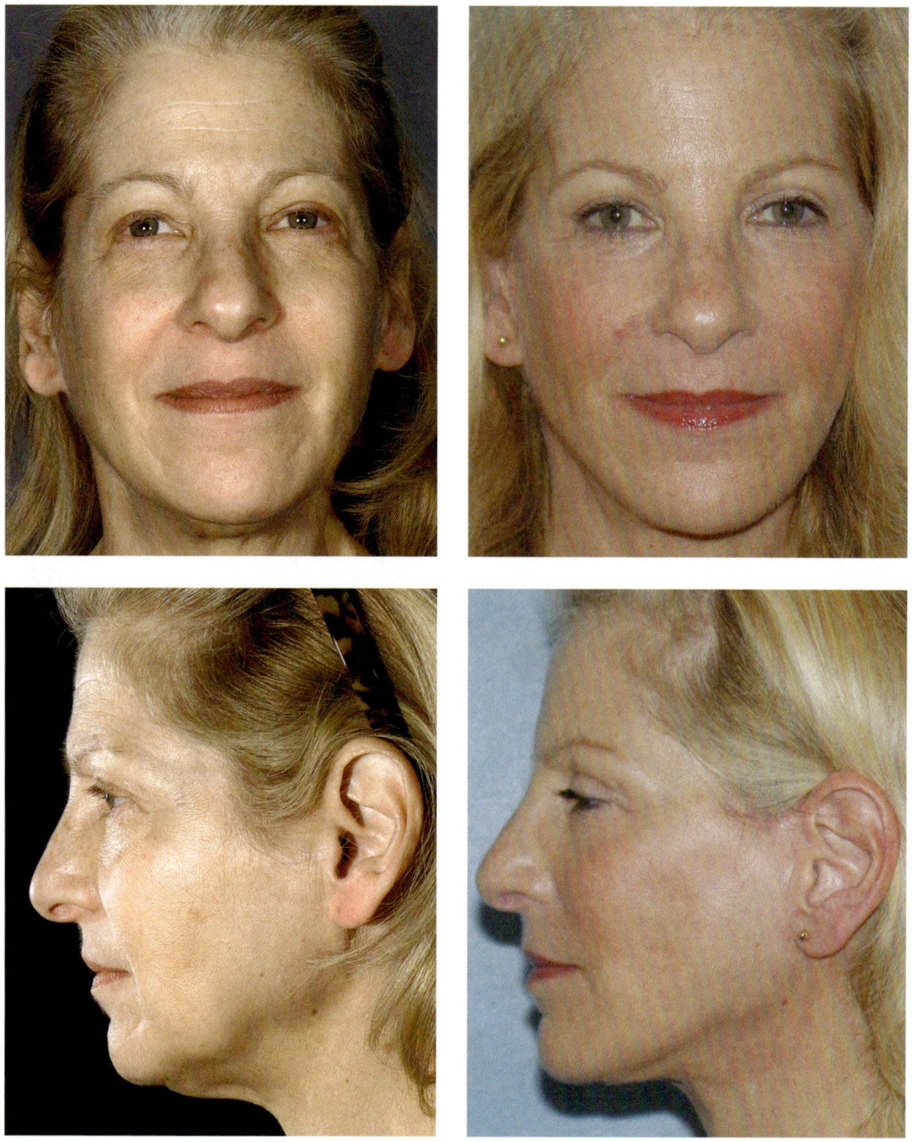

This is a 64-year-old woman who underwent a short scar facelift, submentalplasty, and upper and transconjunctival lower eyelid. Early postoperative views.

Potential Problems and Complications

Application of the glue without the aerosolized sprayer may cause clumping and deposition of too much glue. Evenly spraying the glue on the flap and raw surfaces prevents pooling of the product, which can lead to improper coaptation of the flaps. Timing of glue application is important to prevent improper redraping. Application of glue early without complete flap redraping may cause incorrect redraping and improper vectors on the flaps. Finally, the glue is not a substitute for meticulous hemostasis and will not stop arterial bleeding or vigorous venous bleeding.

The short scar facelift may cause temporary bunching in the temporal and postauricular regions that should be adjusted intraoperatively, although small residual bunching quickly resolves. The short scar incision does not provide access to the temporal region. Also, in patients with severely damaged neck skin, it does not allow excessive "pulling" or "tightening," which, however, we do not believe would compensate for the damaged collagen and elastin that is the etiology of the problem. Rather, a process that theoretically improves the damaged skin, such as topical chemicals or nonablative lasers, radiofrequency systems, or intense pulse light therapy, would be more appropriate.

Hematomas are the most common complication of facelift surgery and occur in from 4% to 15% of patients.[18] In our series of 427 consecutive patients, none of the final 188 patients who were treated with tissue glue experienced hematoma or seroma formation requiring reoperation. There were cases of smaller fluid collections requiring needle aspiration in the office. Hematoma formation can lead to tissue ischemia, prolonged facial edema, hyperpigmentation, reoperation, and patient dissatisfaction. Traditionally the use of vacuum drains has been recommended to diminish fluid collections and "reduce" the incidence of hematoma formation postoperatively.[19] Drains, however, are associated with morbidity, which may include infection, tracts at the site of drain removal, painful extraction, the possibility of injury to a vessel upon drain removal, and the increased nursing care required for drains. At present the use of drains is often advised; however, based on our experience, the adjunctive use of fibrin sealant in short scar facelift surgery appears to eliminate the need for routine drainage in facelift surgery.

Other studies corroborate these findings. One randomized, double-blind trial of 20 patients compared the drain output after unilateral application of fibrin sealant and the contralateral application of placebo during bilateral facelift. Although no patient incurred the complication of hematoma or seroma, the average drainage on the treated side was 10 ml, significantly less than the control side, which drained an average of 30 ml.[14] Other retrospective studies of patients who underwent rhytidectomy, half with and half without the adjunctive use of fibrin glue, revealed significantly less postoperative ecchymosis and hematoma formation despite the omission of drains and compressive dressings and more rapid recovery in the fibrin glue treatment arms.[8,20]

In this series of 427 consecutive short scar facelift patients, complications included the following:

- Two cases of preauricular skin ischemia (among the first 40 patients who did not have fibrin sealant)
- Two temporary cervical nerve branch injuries (resolved within 6 months)
- Five scar revisions (3 sideburns, 2 post-lobule)
- One deep venous thrombosis/pulmonary embolism (in a patient undergoing multiple face and body procedures)
- Five patients with firm, indurated anterior platysmorrhaphy fullness necessitating treatment

Key Points to Consider in Using Fibrin Sealant

- Education of operating room staff and surgical assistant to the sequence of events using the sealant
- Advance planning for preparation of the product
- Proper mixing of the solution
- Appropriate time of introduction of the solution
- Recommended dividing of the 2 ml among the two halves of the face (0.75 ml per side) and the submental region (0.5 ml)
- Thin, evenly applied layer utilizing the spray application device
- Aerosolization over 1 minute followed by application of continuous pressure for 3 minutes
- Standard hemostasis
- Elimination of the need for vacuum drains

Conclusion: Our Approach to the Use of Tissue Glues in the Short Scar Transauricular Rhytidectomy (5-STAR)

The short scar facelift allows all facelift patients to avoid any hair-bearing incisions; consequently alopecia and hairline abnormalities are eliminated, as are thickened mastoid scars and certain other flap problems. This has resulted in a high degree of patient acceptance. The shift away from a traditional, larger incision to a short incision for all patients is an example of how reconsidering time-honored dogma can change longstanding medical practice (i.e., a short incision was only useful in younger patients). The use of Tisseel fibrin glue has enhanced the efficacy of the procedure by reducing fluid collections, shortening the recovery process, eliminating the use of drains, and facilitating flap repositioning. This series demonstrates our results with the short scar facelift in a large series of 427 consecutive patients by the senior author (A.M.). This series includes men and women ranging in age from 34 to 80, and encompasses those undergoing primary, secondary, or more facelifts. Submentalplasty was performed on 282 patients (66%) who underwent the short scar facelift versus 10.6% of facelift procedures performed with the traditional technique. Concomitant aesthetic procedures were performed on 295 (69%) patients. Fibrin sealant aerosolized via a spray application device was done to achieve cost-effective, superior distribution of a critically thin sealant layer in the last 188 consecutive patients. In patients receiving the fibrin sealant, vacuum drains were not placed postoperatively. Although hematomas remain the most common complication after facelift surgery, none of the 188 patients treated with tissue glue in this series of 427 patients experienced hematoma or seroma formation that required a return to the operating room. At present, the use of drains in facelift surgery remains an unresolved questions; however, based on this and other series[8,14,20] the adjunctive use of fibrin sealant significantly minimizes postoperative bruising, edema, pain, and the risk of hematoma or seroma and apparently also eliminates the need for routine drains in rhytidectomy.

REFERENCES

1. Grey EG. Fibrin as a hemostatic in cranial surgery. Surg Gynecol Obstet 21:452, 1915.
2. Dresdale A, Bowman FO Jr, Malm JR, Reemtsma K, Smith CR, Spotnitz HM, Rose EA. Hemostatic effectiveness of fibrin glue derived from single-donor fresh frozen plasma. Ann Thorac Surg 40:385-387, 1985.
3. Baxter Corporation. Tisseel Vapor Heated Fibrin Sealant. Data on file, Pamphlet 006031, 2002.
4. Bronestedt S, Olson S, Rank F. Wound healing and formation of granulation tissue in normal and defibrinogenated rabbits. Eur Surg Res 10(Suppl 10):104, 1978.
5. Marchac D, Sandor G. Face lifts and sprayed fibrin glue: An outcome analysis of 200 patients. Br J Plast Surg 47:306-309, 1994.
6. Mandel MA. Closure of blepharoplasty incisions with autologous fibrin glue. Arch Ophthalmol 108:842-844, 1990.
7. Marchac D, Ascherman J, Arnaud A. Fibrin glue fixation in forehead endoscopy: Evaluation of our experience with 206 cases. Plast Reconstr Surg 100:704-712, 1997.
8. Matarasso, A. Facialplasty. Dermatol Clin 15:649-658, 1997.
9. Matarasso A, Elkwood A, Rankin M, Elkowitz M. National plastic surgery survey: Face lift techniques and complications. Plast Reconstr Surg 106:1185-1195, 2000. (Cited in Year Book of Plastic and Aesthetic Surgery. St. Louis: Mosby–Year Book, 2002).
10. Nahai F, Feldman J. Personal communication, 2000.
11. Dorner F. Validation of virus removal and inactivation in the course of the manufacture of sealer protein concentrate (human) vapor heated, deficient in factor VIII, using HIV-1, HAV, and model viruses. A Preclinical Study, Internal Study No PR099403, August 22, 1996.
12. Mannucci PM, Schimpf K, Abe T, Aledort LM, Anderle K, Brettler DB, Hilgartner MW, Kernoff PB, Kunschok M, McMillan CW. Low risk of viral infection after administration of vapor-heated factor VIII concentrate. Transfusion 32:134-138, 1992.
13. Nowotny R, Chalupka A, Nowotny C, et al. Mechanical properties of fibrinogen adhesive material. In Winter GD, Gibbons DF, Plank H Jr, eds. Biomaterials. New York: John Wiley & Sons, 1982.
14. Redl H, Schlag G. Properties of different tissue sealants with special emphasis on fibrinogen-based preparations. In Schlag G, Redl H, eds. Fibrin Sealant in Operative Medicine, General Surgery, and Abdominal Surgery, vol. 6. Berlin: Springer-Verlag, 1986.
15. Oliver DW, Hamilton SA, Figle AA, Wood SH, Lamberty BG. A prospective, randomized, double-blind trial of the use of fibrin sealant for face lifts. Plast Reconstr Surg 108:2101-2105, 2001.
16. Kjaergard HK, Trumball HR. Vivostat system autologous fibrin sealant: Preliminary study in elective coronary bypass grafting. Ann Thorac Surg 66:482-486, 1998.
17. Man D, Plosker H, Winland-Brown JE. The use of autologous platelet-rich plasma (platelet gel) and autologous platelet-poor plasma (fibrin glue) in cosmetic surgery. Plast Reconstr Surg 107:229-237, 2001.
18. Baker T, Gordon H. Complications of rhytidectomy. Plast Reconstr Surg 40:31-39, 1967.
19. Perkins SW, Williams JD, Macdonald K, Robinson EB. Prevention of seromas and hematomas after facelift surgery with the use of postoperative vacuum drains. Arch Otolaryngol Head Neck Surg 123:743-745, 1997.
20. Fezza JP, Cartwright M, Mack W, Flaharty P. The use of aerosolized fibrin glue in facelift surgery. Plast Reconstr Surg 110:658-664, 2002.

CHAPTER

9

USE OF FIBRIN TISSUE SEALANT IN FACE AND NECK SURGERY

Barry E. DiBernardo, M.D. ▪ Alfred T. Mitchell, M.D. ▪
Robert B. Nemerofsky, M.D.

Aesthetic surgery today encompasses a wide spectrum of procedures and technologies, allowing improvement in form, cutaneous texture, and laxity, yet there is a continued pursuit of less involved procedures, shorter recovery time, and improved results.

The use of fibrin tissue sealants in aesthetic surgery has increased, particularly in facial applications. Inherent in many of these surgical procedures is the separation of the skin from underlying structures, creating a potential space. In the postoperative healing period this space is vulnerable to collections of serum or blood that produce prolonged swelling, ecchymosis, and possible unevenness in the final healing. If this space is excessive, seromas or hematomas can result, necessitating postoperative intervention. In the past we have tried to close these potential spaces by suctioning them and applying pressure dressings, both of which increase the complexity of the patient's postoperative course. It is the function of the sealant to "close" or diminish this potential space within minutes of application, therefore reducing the healing-phase stigmas and potential complications in the postoperative period. Patients can resume normal activities faster, which is the objective in both facial surgical and laser-based treatments.

In addition to the benefits in the immediate postoperative period, there are long-term benefits to using fibrin sealants in the face and neck. Beyond a certain age, in the mid-thirties, fibroblasts reduce their production of elastin. The laxity and reduced elasticity of the skin becomes progressively worse with age. Because the older population is more likely to undergo facial procedures, areas below the mandible have to conform to the underlying muscle against gravity. Again it is the added immediate structural support of the fibrin network that holds this skin in position early, leading to an improved long-term result.

TABLE 9-1 POTENTIAL BENEFIT OF TISSUE SEALANTS WITH SURGICAL APPROACHES FOR SIX TYPES OF PATIENTS

Patient Type	Age	Skin Laxity and Elasticity	Neck Fat	Neck Muscle Laxity/Ptosis	Cheek Muscle Laxity/Jowls	Quantity Glue (ml)
I	Younger	+	−	+	+	1
II	Younger	+	−	−	+	1
III	Younger	+	±	−	+	1
IV	Younger/older	−	±	−	+	2
V	Younger/older	−	±	+	−	2
VI	Older	−	±	−	−	2

+ = Beneficial; − = Not beneficial.

INDICATIONS FOR USE

Fibrin tissue sealants are indicated for any potential space or separation of skin of the face or neck. Depending on the variables of age—skin laxity and elasticity, distribution of fat, muscle laxity, and neck contour—one of six surgical approaches is used. The potential benefit of the use of fibrin sealant with each type of surgery is indicated in Table 9-1.

Age is a factor in the general appreciation of skin and muscle laxity. Younger patients usually require less intervention because their skin tone is good. Excess adipose tissue is usually the focus of the contour complaint. The range of procedure and therefore the amount of sealant indicated increases with the extent of undermining. Cervical fat, cheek and neck laxity, and skin quality are evaluated by physical examination. Specific readings of skin laxity and elasticity can be evaluated by the BTC-2000 to obtain quantitative readings of these parameters directly.

Patients are grouped into one of the following six categories:

Type I: Neck Suction-Assisted Lipoplasty (SAL) + Glue

Type I is a younger patient with good skin quality and muscle tone but excess fat. Although liposuction of the neck has been adequate in the past, the addition of fibrin sealant has closed the space, enhanced skin adherence, and reduced swelling in this procedure.

Type II: Neck SAL + Anterior Muscle Plication + Glue

Type II is a younger patient as in type I; however, once fat is removed, the ideal neck contour is hampered by loose muscle. Therefore the neck is suctioned, anterior platysmal plication is performed, and tissue glue is applied.

Type III: Neck Suture Suspension 2 + Glue

Type III patient is as described for type II except that excess adipose tissue may not be the primary problem; there is more muscle laxity and neck ptosis. A more obtuse cervicomental angle is present with possibly platysmal banding as well. The patient also desires an enhanced jaw line.

Type IV: Neck Suture Suspension + Extended Posterior Skin Excision + Glue

In type IV the neck has good contour and muscle tone. Complaints are restricted to jowling or prominence of the nasolabial folds. There is cheek laxity in both skin and underlying musculature. A superficial musculoaponeurotic system (SMAS) plication or partial excision is performed addressing excess skin; 1 ml of fibrin sealant is used on each side, for a total of 2 ml.

Type V: Temporal or Mid-Face Rhytidectomy (Cheek Only) + Glue

Type V patients are older, with skin laxity, loss of elasticity, and poor muscle tone; 2 ml of sealant is divided equally among the right and left sides of the face.

Type VI: Rhytidectomy (Cheek and Neck) + Glue

Type VI patients exhibit the same symptoms as those in type V. In addition, they also have jowling and neck ptosis; 2 ml of sealant is divided equally among the right and left sides of the face and the neck.

Preparation of Material

Because the thrombin is responsible for the setting time of the fibrin sealant, it is possible to lengthen the setting time by diluting the thrombin 500 IU/ml to 5 IU/ml (see box on p. 153). The fibrin sealant will start to set within 30 to 60 seconds after spray application, allowing time for manipulation and postioning of the skin flaps.

The resulting 2 ml of solution (5 IU/ml of thrombin) is now in the small black vial and is ready to be drawn up to the field. The Fibrinotherm device (Baxter Corporation, Deerfield, Ill.) (Fig. 9-1, *A*) is used for reconstitution of the fibrin sealant along with the Tissomat and spray set device (Baxter Corporation) (Fig. 9-1, *B*) for delivery of aerosolized fibrin glue.

Instructions for Diluting Thrombin 500 IU/ml to 5 IU/ml to Delay Clot Formation

Dilution of Tisseel 2 ml Kit

One vial of 0.9% sodium chloride (10 ml) with *no* preservatives is also needed.
Use the **same black-scaled syringe** throughout this process.

1. Reconstitute the sealer protein (blue vial) as usual.
2. Using the ***black-scaled*** syringe, draw up ***1 ml*** $\boldsymbol{CaCl_2}$ from the ***small black vial*** and discard it.
3. Draw up ***2 ml NaCl*** and inject it into the ***thrombin*** vial: it will dissolve the thrombin completely.
4. Draw up ***0.2 ml*** of this reconstituted thrombin solution.
5. Add ***1.8 ml NaCl*** (2 ml of solution total); rotate syringe to mix components.
6. Discard ***1.8 ml*** (0.2 ml remaining).
7. Add ***0.8 ml NaCl*** (1 ml of solution total).
8. Inject this 1 ml of solution into the $\boldsymbol{CaCl_2}$ ***vial.***
9. Label this small black vial as ***thrombin 5 IU/ml.***

A

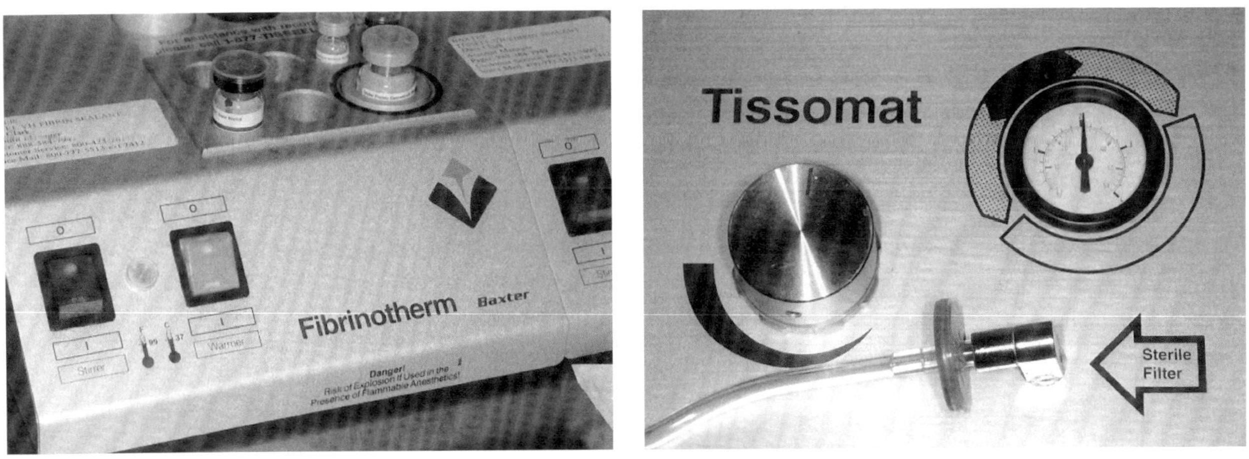

B

Figure 9-1 **A,** Fibrinotherm device. **B,** Tissomat and spray set device.

Timing in Use of Materials

The Tisseel VH kit (Baxter Corporation) contains all the components necessary for the preparation of fibrin sealant. There are four vials in each kit: a sealer protein, a fibrinolysis inhibitor solution, thrombin, and calcium chloride solution (Fig. 9-2, *A*). Preparation of the glue involves heating the sealer protein and the fibrinolysis inhibitor for 10 to 15 minutes in the Fibrinotherm device (see Fig. 9-1, *A*) and then mixing them to form the sealer protein solution. The thrombin and calcium chloride are combined to form a thrombin solution. Two components, the protein sealant and thrombin solution, are then placed in separate syringes in the dual injection system (Duploject applicator) (Fig. 9-2, *B*), which allows equal amounts of these key ingredients to be delivered to the tissue. The dual syringe is connected to the spray device and Tissomat (Fig. 9-2, *C*), a pressurized nitrogen gas tank, which aerosolizes the glue into a fine mist. This allows for delivery of a thin layer of glue evenly to the tissues and avoids clumping of the sealant. Once reconstituted, the sealer protein and the thrombin solutions must be used within 4 hours. If more than 4 hours pass before the reconstituted solutions are used, the solutions must not be used and should be disposed of properly.

Application of Tissue Glue

The reconstituted sealer protein vial and thrombin vial remain warm in the Fibrinotherm device at a temperature of 37° C (see Fig. 9-1, *A*). To ensure homogeneity, the magnetic stirrer of the Fibrinotherm device is switched on shortly before the solution is drawn up. The protein sealant and thrombin solution are then placed in separate syringes in the dual injection system (Duploject applicator) (see Fig. 9-2, *B*), which allows equal amounts of these key ingredients to be delivered to the tissue. The dual syringe is connected to the Tissomat and spray set device (see Fig. 9-2, *C*), a pressurized system that aerosolizes the glue into a fine mist. This allows for delivery of a thin layer of glue evenly to the tissue. A 2 ml kit is used for each facelift (1 ml glue per side).

A

B

C

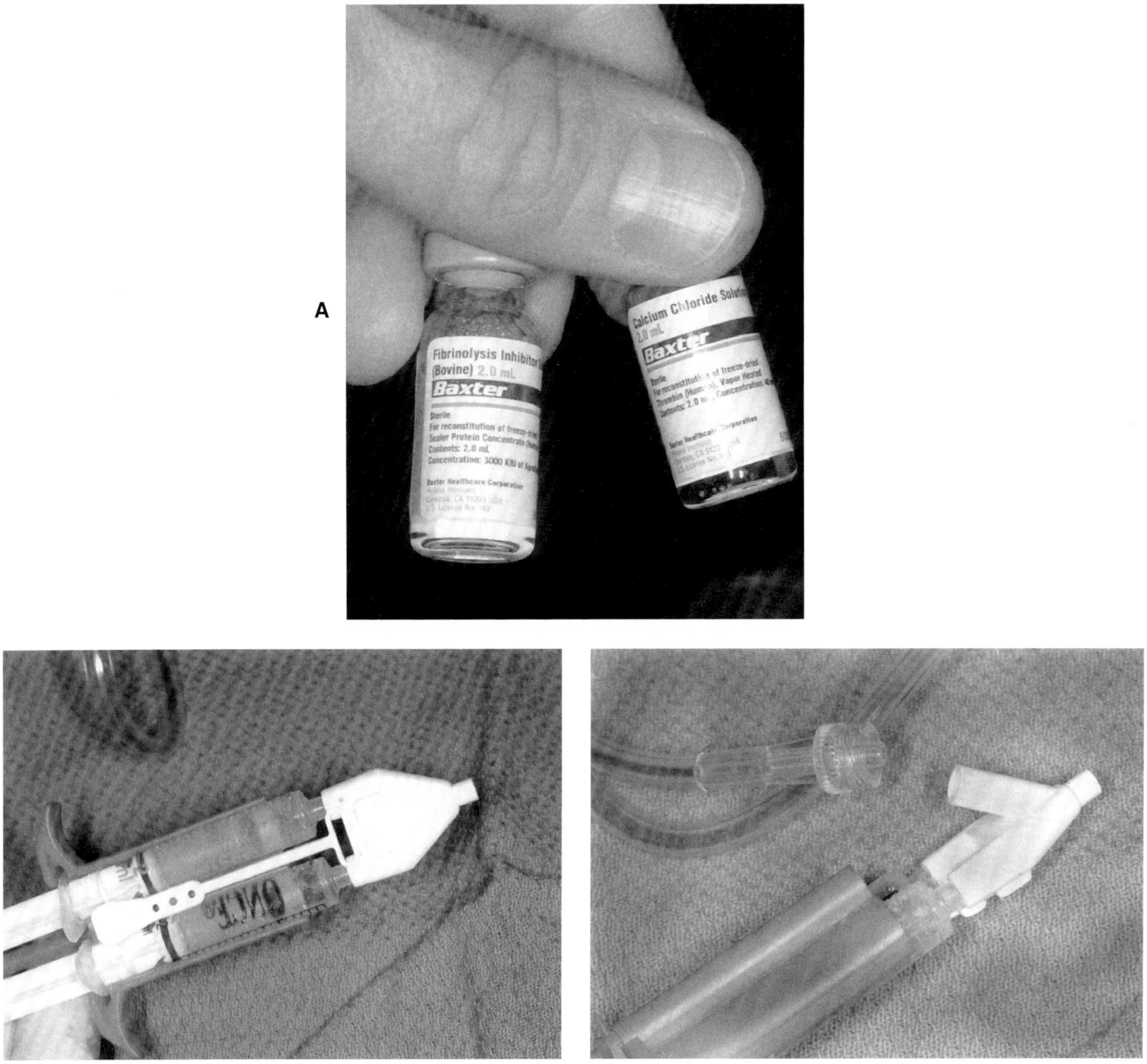

Figure 9-2 **A,** Calcium chloride solution and fibrinolysis inhibitor solution. **B,** Duploject applicator. **C,** Duploject applicator and spray set device.

Preparation of Wound

After elevation of the skin flaps, heavy bleeding must be controlled and meticulous hemostasis achieved before the aerosolized fibrin sealant is applied. The skin flaps are trimmed, and key points are marked along the preauricular and postauricular region to assist with closure of the skin (Fig. 9-3, *A* and *B*). The Tissomat and spray set device are also used to optimize adherence and sealing by drying the wound surface with compressed gas before the fibrin glue is applied.

Surgical Technique

Our approach to rhytidectomies and platysmaplasty with suture suspension technique is performed with the patient under general anesthesia, although local anesthesia can be used. Preoperatively the proposed incision lines are drawn with a surgical marker. We use a standard rhytidectomy and submental incision. The temporal incision is placed within the hairline, beginning at a point immediately superior to the junction of the ear with the temporal skin. The preauricular segment of the incision follows the posterior margin of the tragus and inferiorly contours the margins of the earlobe. The postauricular incision is placed directly within the conchal groove and then is extended into the hairline where the concha joins the hairline. Lidocaine 1% with epinephrine 1:100,000 is infiltrated along the proposed incision lines, and a 0.5% lidocaine solution with 1:400,000 epinephrine is infiltrated into the anticipated plane of dissection.

The dissection is started on the right side in the temporal region. After the skin is incised, the dissection is continued through the temporoparietal fascia down to the loose areolar tissue overlying the deep temporal fascia. A combination of sharp and blunt dissection, often using gentle finger dissection, assists with development of this plane. The dissection within the cheek is carried subcutaneously superficial to the SMAS. Care must be taken to protect the frontal branch of the facial nerve in the transition zone between the temporal region and the cheek. The postauricular dissection is carried just superficial to the fascia overlying the sternocleidomastoid muscle. As the dissection proceeds caudal to the level of the earlobe, it becomes more superficial and is carried through the subcutaneous fat to protect the underlying great auricular nerve.

Once the skin flap has been elevated and hemostasis achieved, markings are made on the SMAS. Using a small rake, laxity in the SMAS is evaluated, which will determine placement of SMAS plication sutures (Fig. 9-3, *C*). Markings are placed at the upper and lower pole for SMAS plication. The SMAS plication is performed with 3-0 clear nylon sutures.

These buried interrupted sutures are placed through the area. Excess skin is evaluated and trimmed with a No. 15 scalpel blade (see Fig. 9-3, *A*). The surgeon then turns to the submental region. A curvilinear submental incision is made, and the skin immediately overlying the platysma muscle in its midline is elevated with facelift scissors. Redundant fatty tissue immediately overlying the platysma muscle is suctioned with a 4 mm spatula cannula. The submental skin and neck below the area of dissection and the lateral neck skin are also suctioned with a 4 mm spatula cannula. The area of the submandibular tunnel is suctioned along its dermal surface.

The platysma border in the midline is usually resected and the borders cauterized to control bleeding. The midline of the platysma is sutured with buried mattress 3-0 Prolene sutures to reapproximate and, in effect, shorten the width

A

B

C

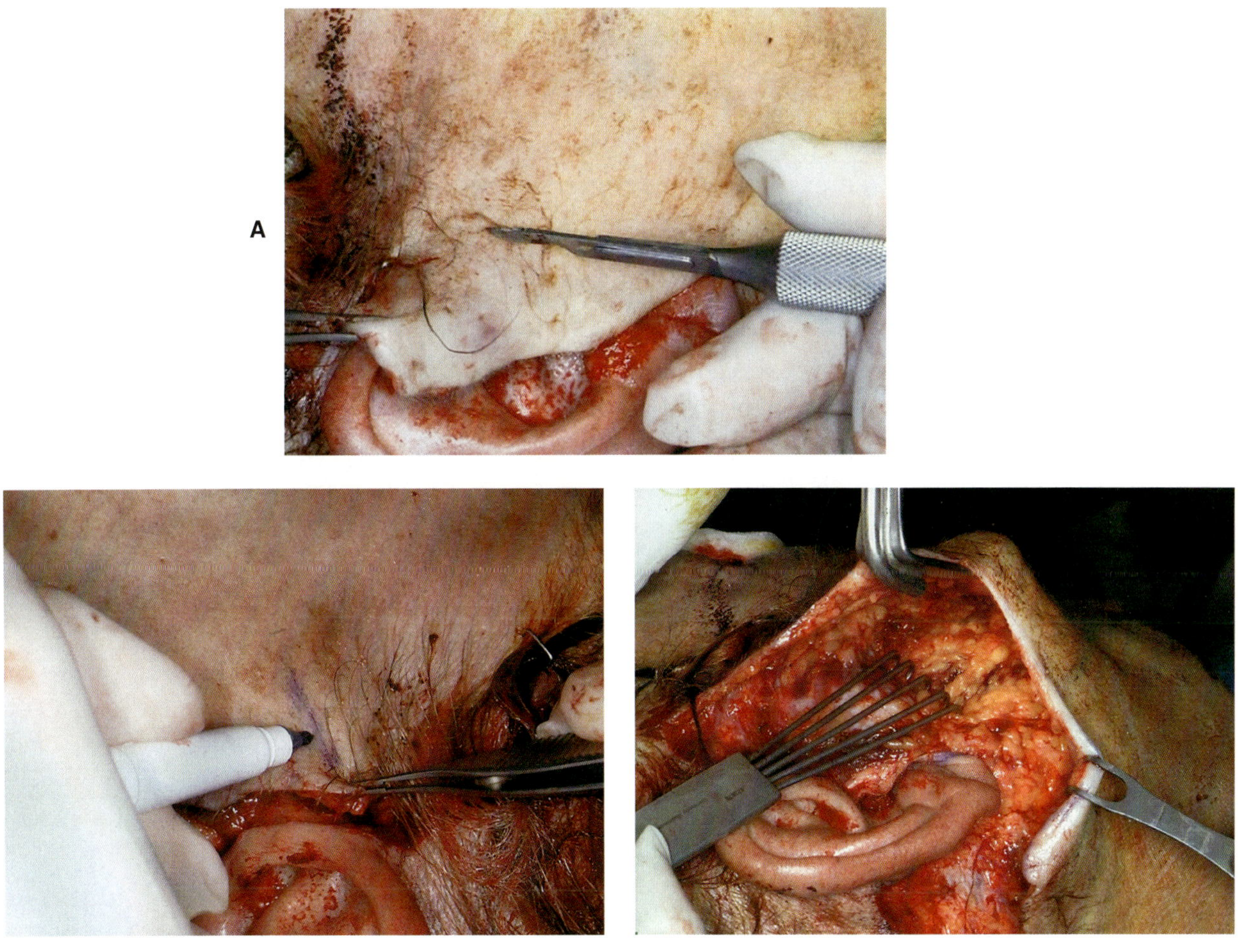

Figure 9-3 **A,** Excision of excess skin, preauricular auricular areas. **B,** Key points marked along the preauricular and auricular areas. **C,** Evaluation of superficial musculoaponeurotic system laxity. *Continued.*

of the platysma muscle. At the depth desired to create the new cervicomental angle, 3-0 Prolene sutures are placed in horizontal mattress fashion from right to left, including both borders of the platysma muscle (Fig. 9-3, *D*). Then a suture is placed from left to right in a vertical mattress style, interlocking with the first suture. The ends of both sutures are taken out through the submental incision, and the sutures are clamped separately with a needle holder. A long, curved hemostat is placed behind the postauricular sulcus and exits through the tunnel at the submental incision. The right suture is grasped in the instrument and taken through the submandibular tunnel. A horizontal mattress suture is passed deep into the mastoid fascia (Fig. 9-3, *E*). The suture is then tied just enough so the platysma muscle is tucked up underneath the border of the mandible. This skin can be seen under direct vision. The skin contracts, with a sudden definition appearing below the submandibular border. A similar procedure is carried out on the contralateral side.

The fibrin tissue sealant is mixed while the dissection is being performed. Once the fibrin sealant is ready for injection, the spray tubing is placed to aerosolize the tissue glue. After careful hemostasis is achieved, the fibrin tissue sealant is sprayed in a thin layer on the undermined areas under the skin flap (Fig. 9-3, *F*). We use 2 ml of fibrin glue divided among the right and left cheeks and anterior neck. One minute is allotted to spray the glue and to secure the premarked areas with staples anteriorly and posteriorly. Compression is then placed on the face and neck for 3 minutes by the clock. After 3 minutes the areas are inspected for adherence of the skin to the underlying structures and closure of the potential space (Fig. 9-3, *G*). The glue is then applied to the submental region in the potential space, the incision is stapled closed, and light compression is applied throughout the neck region for 3 minutes (Fig. 9-3, *H* to *J*). A similar procedure is carried out on the contralateral side.

D

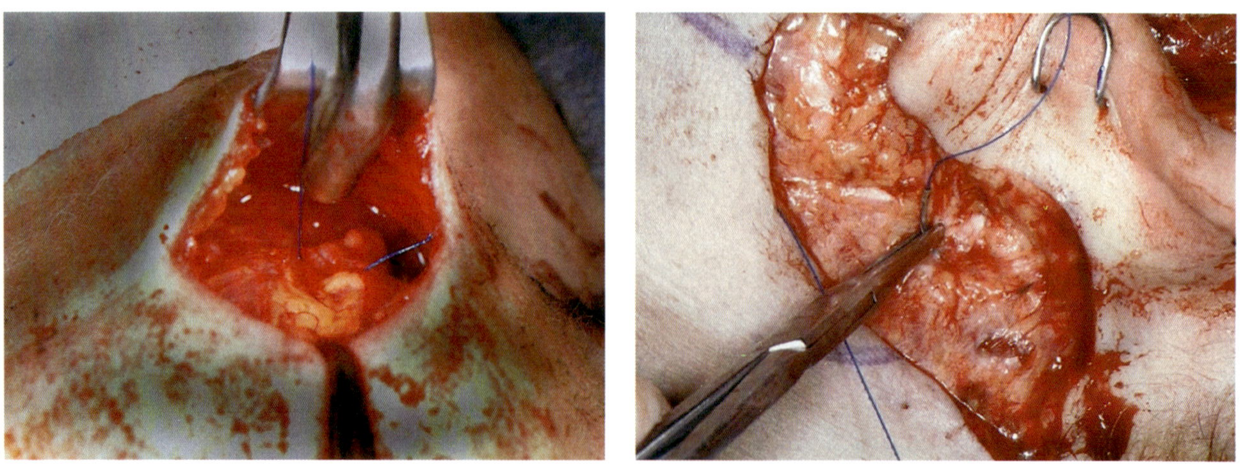

E

Figure 9-3, cont'd **D,** 3-0 Prolene interlocking suspension suture. **E,** Horizontal mattress suture in the mastoid fascia.

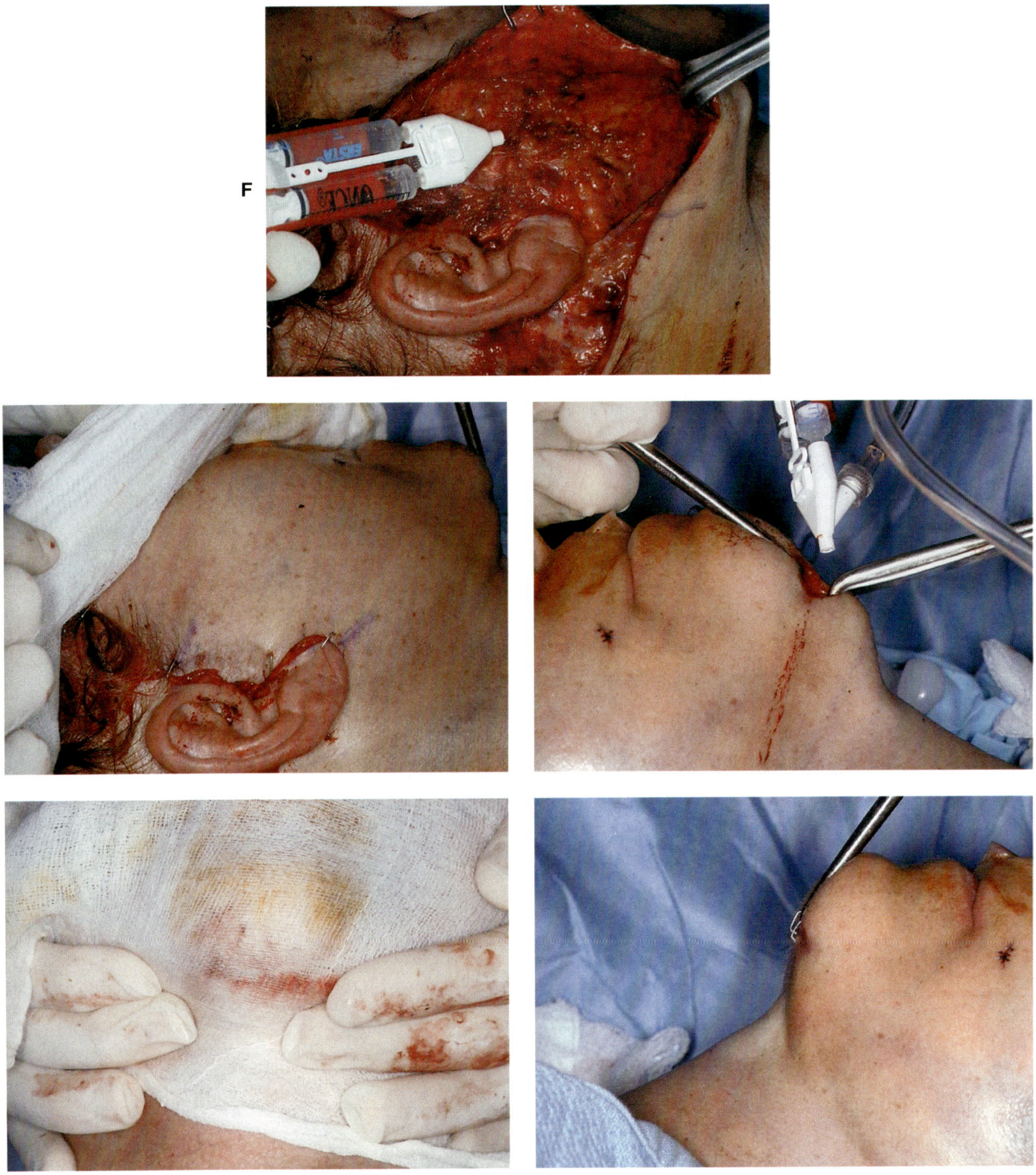

Figure 9-3, cont'd F, Thin layer of fibrin glue sprayed on the undermined area. **G,** Inspection of skin adherence following application of fibrin glue. **H,** Fibrin glue applied to the submental area. **I,** Light compression is applied along the neck and submental areas. **J,** After application of fibrin glue to the submental and neck areas.

Case Examples

Three cases illustrate the use of fibrin glue in a type VI rhytidectomy (cheek and neck).

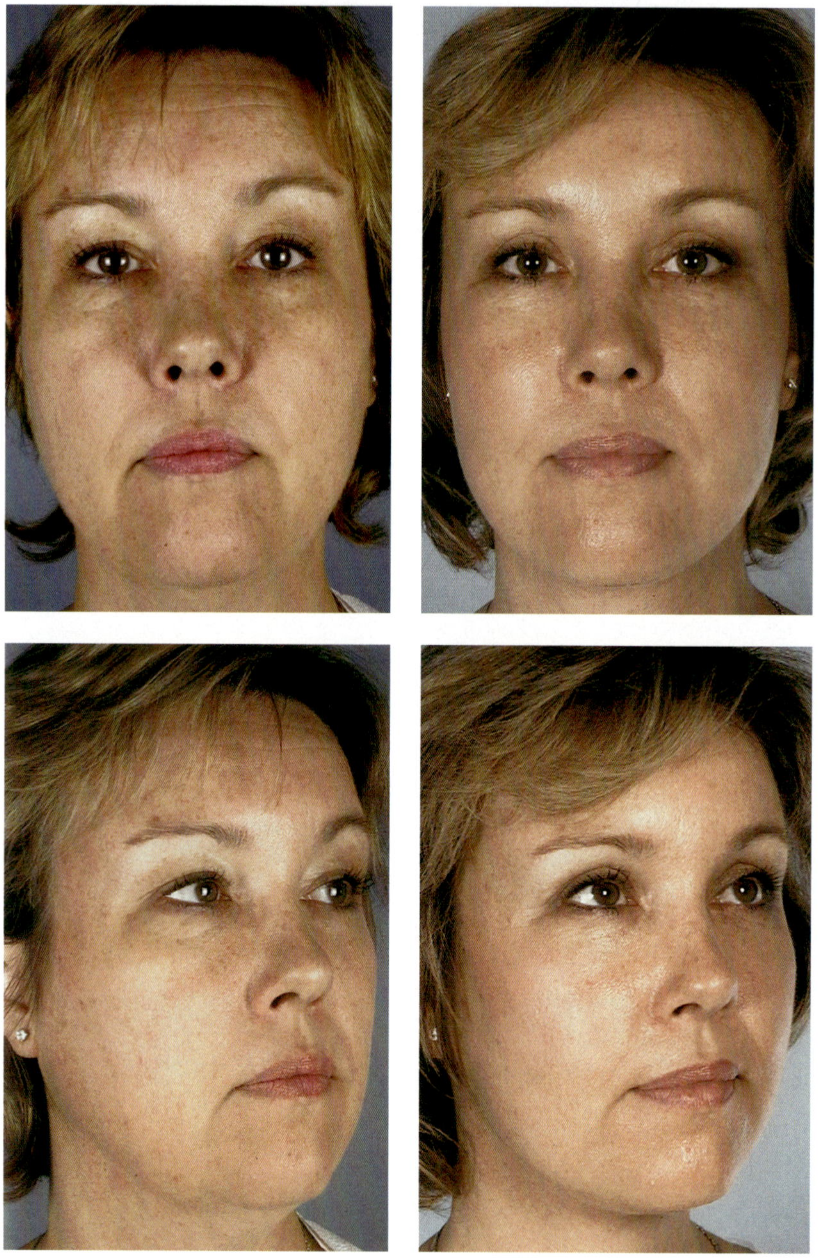

This 49-year-old woman exhibited moderately severe laxity of the skin and platysma muscle. Results are shown 3 weeks after blepharoplasty, rhytidectomy, and suture suspension platysmaplasty.

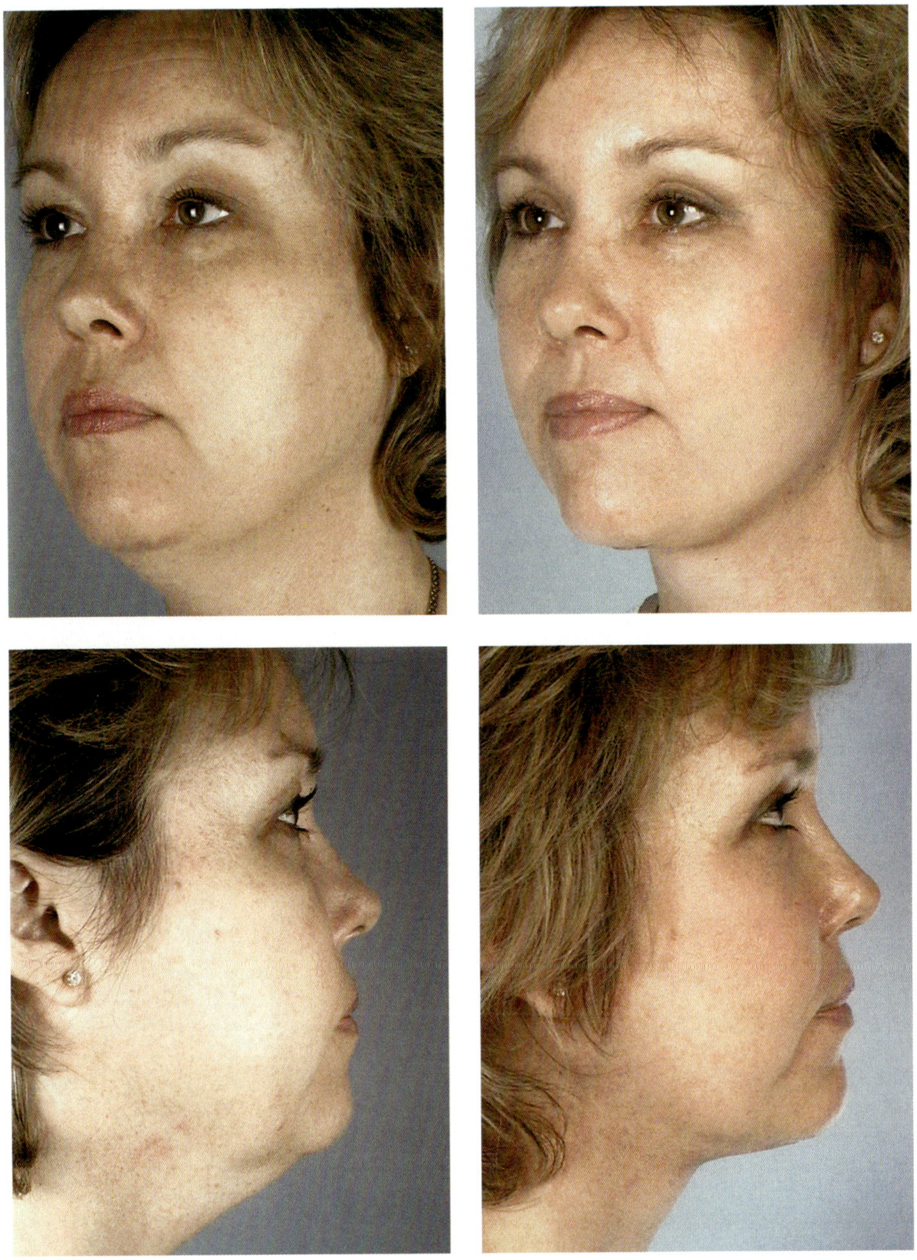

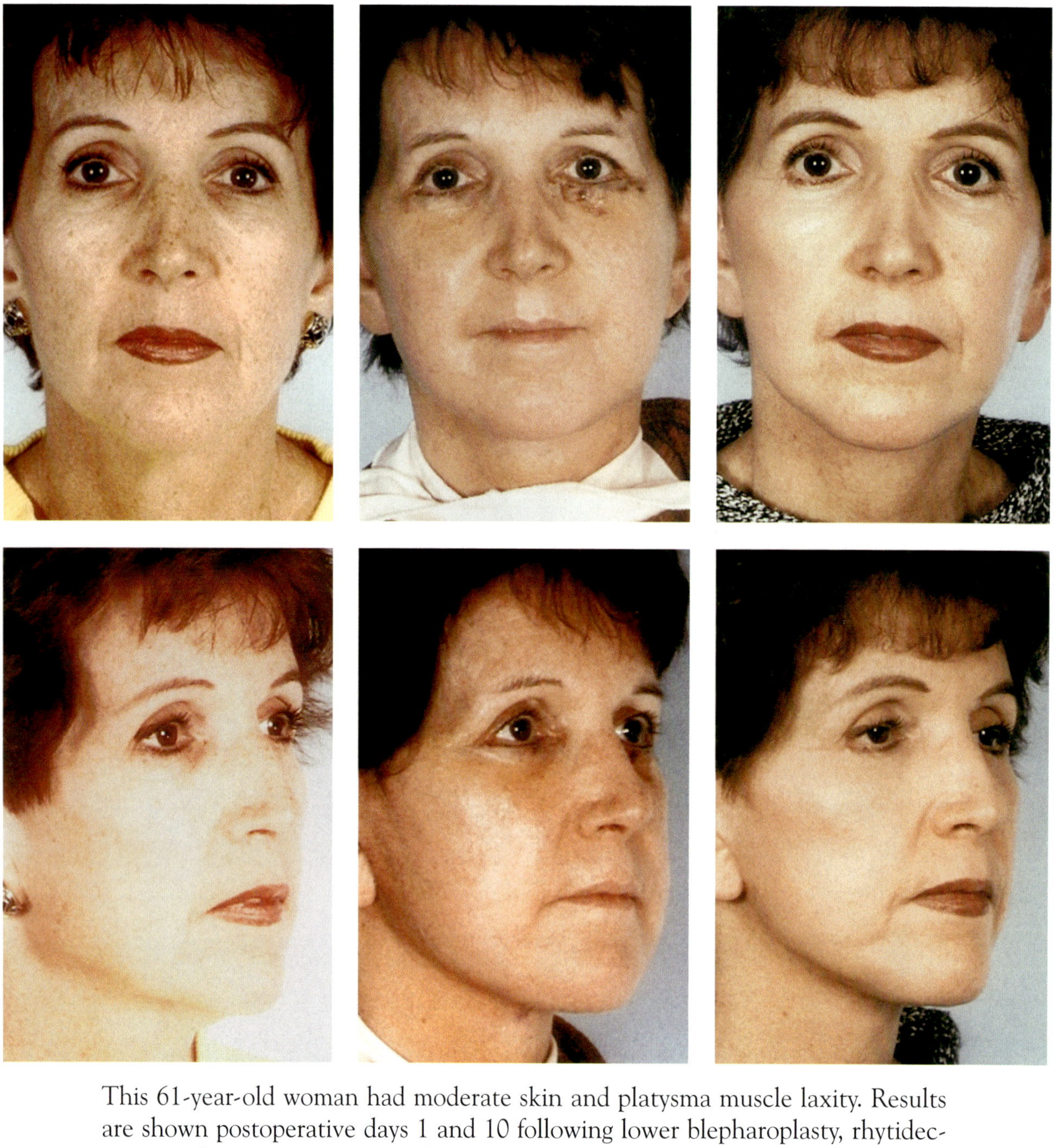

This 61-year-old woman had moderate skin and platysma muscle laxity. Results are shown postoperative days 1 and 10 following lower blepharoplasty, rhytidectomy, and suture suspension platysmaplasty with fibrin glue.

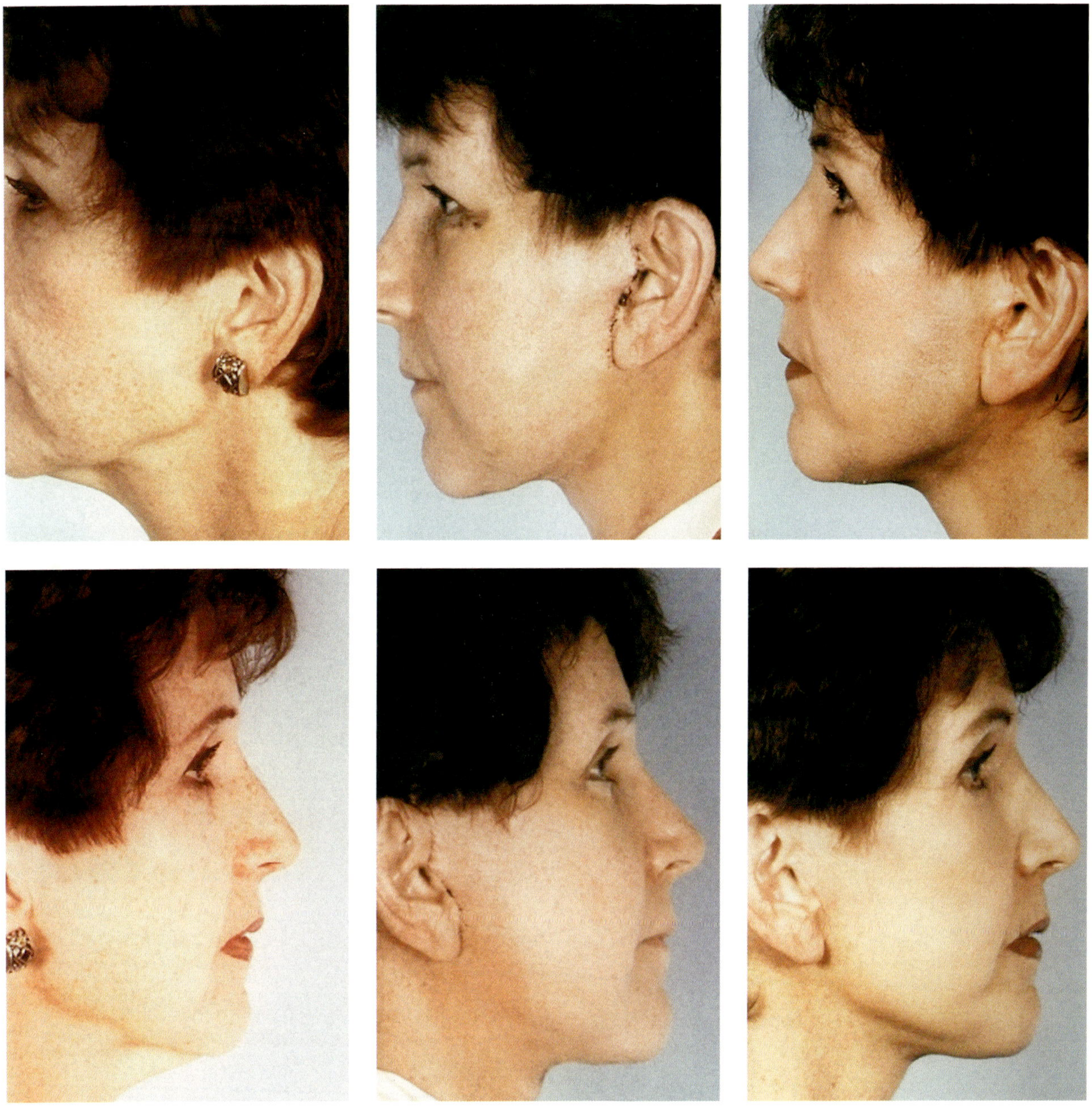

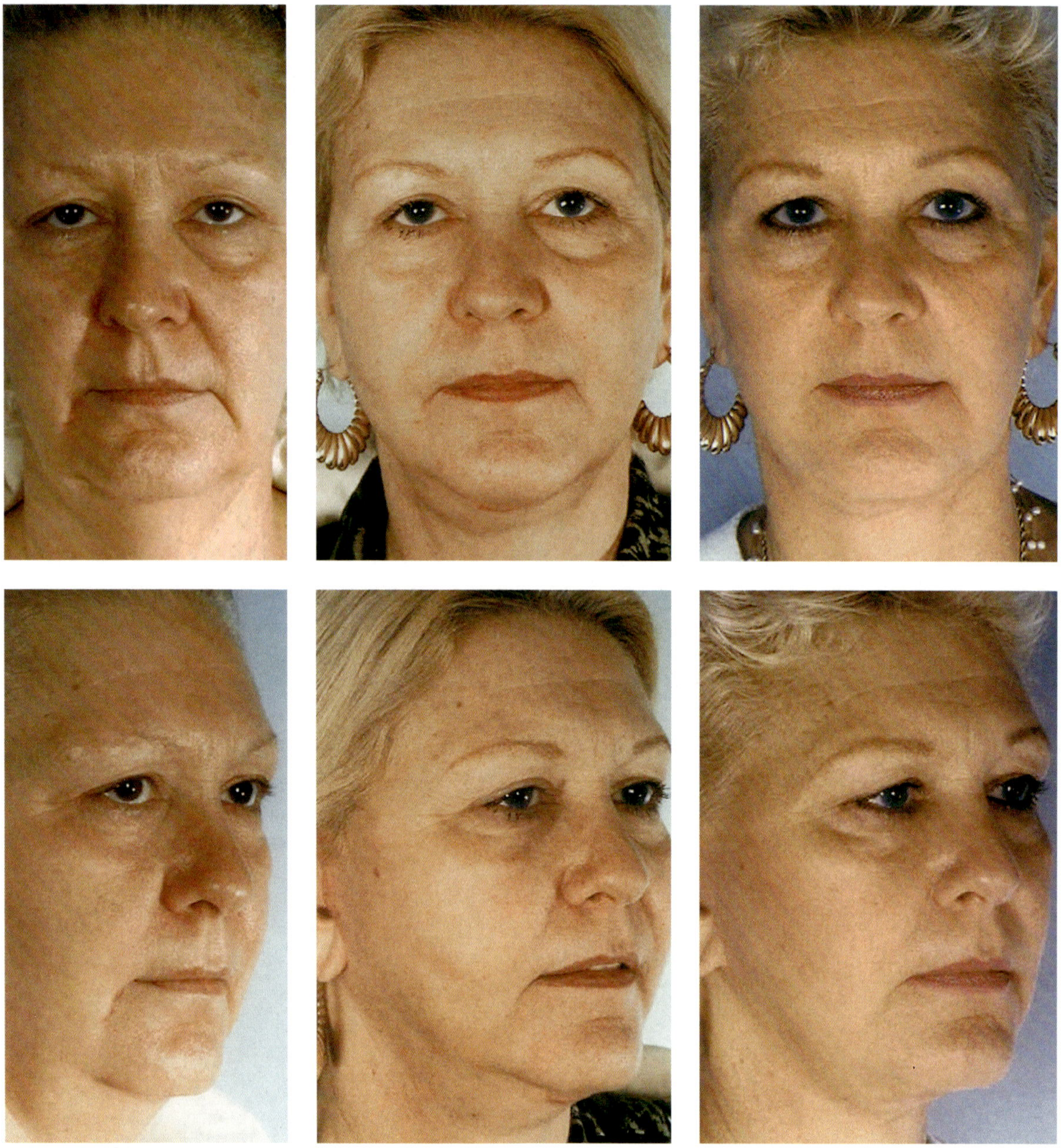

This 56-year-old woman presented with severe skin and platysma muscle laxity. Results are shown 1 year after rhytidectomy and suture suspension without fibrin glue. Results are also shown 1 year after a secondary rhytidectomy and suture suspension with fibrin glue.

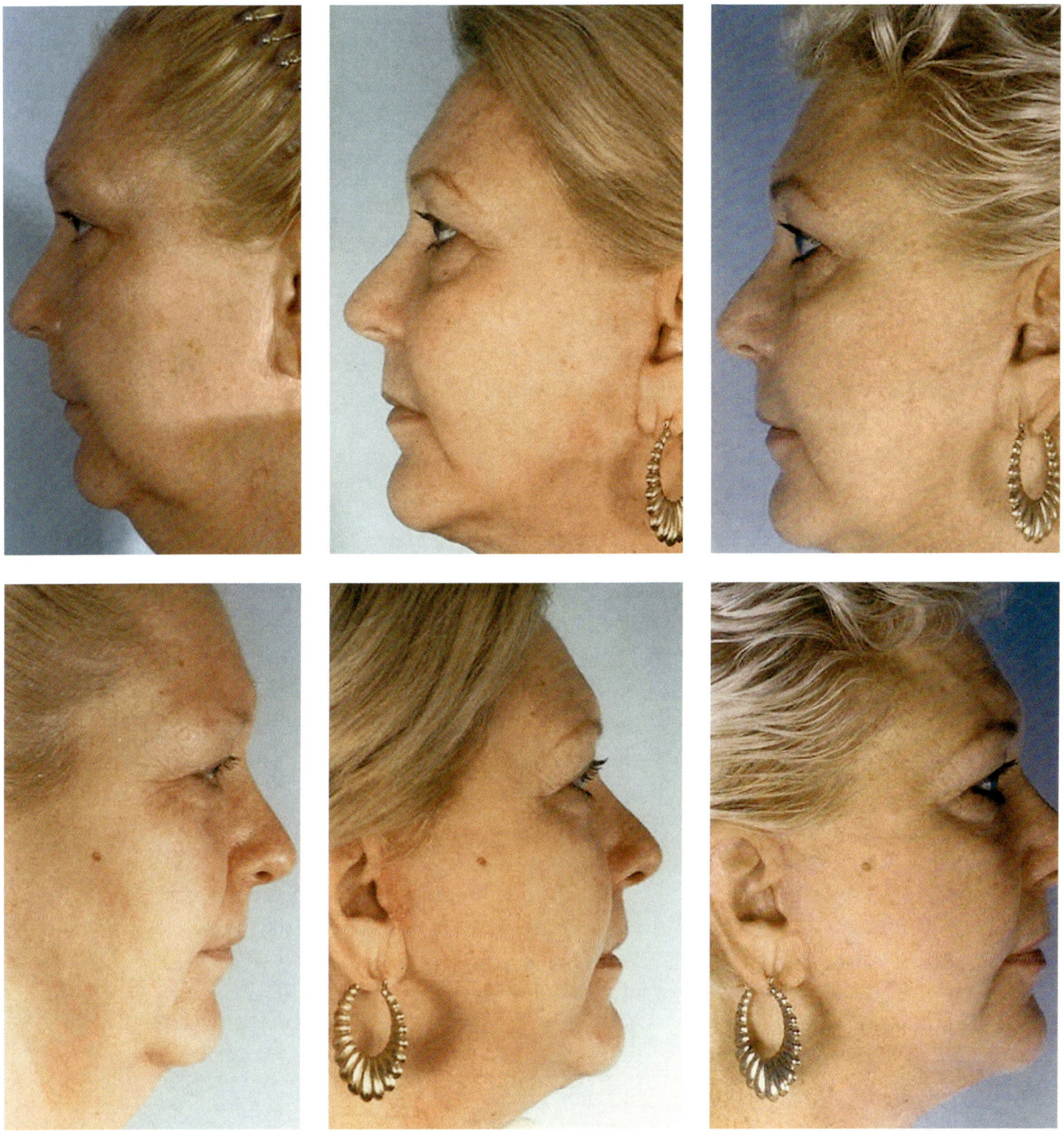

Problems, Pitfalls, and Potential Complications

- Hematomas
- Trapped air pockets
- Infection
- Edema
- Scars
- Ecchymosis

Key Points to Consider When Using Tissue Glues

- Mixing of the fibrin glue must be precise.
- Meticulous hemostasis is essential.
- The skin flaps should be trimmed or tailored before application of the glue.
- The key points for skin closure are marked.
- A thin layer of aerosolized fibrin glue is used.
- Light compression is applied for 3 minutes.

Conclusion: Our Approach to the Use of Tissue Glues

When patients are seen for correction of facial aging, a variety of procedures can be offered to improve the appearance of the face and neck. During consultation the addition of tissue glue to the procedure is discussed, emphasizing enhanced recovery, the decreased need for drains, and the fact that the material is derived from human donors. Patients are also given written materials to review. Fewer than 1% of patients have declined its use.

At the time of surgery the glue is prepared and used as described. Rarely do these patients need drains. A compression dressing is applied for the first night; this is changed to a Velcro chin strap the next day. The chin strap is worn frequently in the first weeks and nightly during the second and third weeks. We have used tissue glues in facial cases for the last 2½ years with good patient compliance and success.

Suggested Readings

Bruck HG. Fibrin tissue adhesion and its use in rhytidectomy: A pilot study. Aesthetic Plast Surg 6:197-202, 1982.

Ellis DA, Shaikh A. The ideal tissue adhesive in facial plastic and reconstructive surgery. J Otolaryngol 19:68-72, 1990.

Giampapa VC, DiBernardino BE. Neck recontouring with suture suspension and liposuction: An alternative for early rhytidectomy candidate. Aesthetic Plast Surg 19(3):217-223, 1995.

Gibble JW, Ness PM. Fibrin glue: The perfect operative sealant? Transfusion 30:741-747, 1990.

Lerner R, Binur NS. Current status of surgical adhesives. J Surg Res 48:165-181, 1990.

Marchac D, Pugash E, Gault D. The use of sprayed fibrin glue in facelifts. Eur J Plast Surg 10:139, 1987.
Marchac D, Sandor G. Facelifts and sprayed fibrin glue: An outcome analysis of 200 patients. Br J Plast Surg 47:306-309, 1994.
Martinowtiz U, Spotnitz WD. Fibrin tissue adhesives. Thromb Haemost 78:661-666, 1997.
Oliver DW, Hamilton SA, Figle AA, Wood SH. A prospective, randomized, double-blind trial of the use of fibrin sealants for facelifts. Plast Reconstr Surg 108:2101-2105, 2001.
Saltz R, Sierra D, Feldman D, Saltz M, Dimick A, Vasconez L. Experimental and clinical applications of fibrin glue. Plast Reconstr Surg 88:1005-1015, 1991.
Spotnitz WD. Fibrin sealant in the United States: Clinical use at the University of Virginia. Thromb Haemost 74:482-485, 1995.
Tisseel Fibrin Sealant (package insert). Deerfield, Ill: Baxter Corporation, 2000.

CHAPTER

10

Use of Cyanoacrylate in Breast and Body Contouring

Ricardo C. Ribeiro, M.D. ▪ Ewaldo Bolivar de Souza Pinto, M.D. ▪
Renato Saltz, M.D.

The possibility of avoiding sutures in surgical and traumatic wounds has been a long-standing goal of most surgeons. With the development of biological and nonbiological glues for this purpose, this objective has become a reality. Today tissue adhesive use has been accepted in many surgical specialties. For example, in plastic surgery it has broad applications to many cosmetic and reconstructive procedures such as facelift, browlift, breast surgery, and body contouring surgery.

Tissue glues fall into two basic categories: (1) the biological glues, including fibrin sealants, platelet gels, albumin with adhesive components, the hydrogels, and adhesives based in collagen, and (2) the nonbiological glues represented by the cyanoacrylates.[1] The synthetic glues generally are recommended for external use, especially in approximating the margins in elective surgery or trauma. This chapter focuses on the role of cyanoacrylates in breast and body contouring as effective alternatives to traditional suturing techniques.

History

The cyanoacrylates were introduced to the scientific community in 1949 as a group of monomers that through an exothermic polymerization reaction demonstrates an important adhesive quality when they come in contact with fluids or tissues. In 1959 the first clinical applications were with their primary derivatives: the methyl-2-cyanoacrylate and ethyl-2-cyanoacrylate. These formulations are efficient adhesives; however, their degradation into cyanoacetate and formaldehyde occurs quickly, leading to tissue toxicity. With the accumulation of these by-products, significant acute and chronic inflammatory reactions were observed as well as granulomatosis and necrosis.

The speed of the degradation was related to the length of the alkyl chains. The longer the chain, the slower the degradation, thus promoting more efficient absorption and processing of the toxic by-products by the tissues. The efficient clearing of these by-products resulted in decreased toxicity and less inflammation. Therefore longer chained substances were developed—initially as the

N-butyl-cyanoacrylate (Histoacryl, B. Braun, Melsungen, Germany) and more recently as octyl-2-cyanoacrylate (Dermabond, Ethicon, Somerville, N.Y.).

Octyl-2-cyanoacrylate is effective for superficial skin closure. Plasticizers added to the product have made the adhesive less brittle, more flexible, and with a tensile strength almost equivalent to nylon 5-0 suture.[2,3]

Several studies suggest that octyl-2-cyanoacrylate has an antimicrobial action.[4-6] The impermeability obtained with this product creates an important barrier to microorganism penetration into the wound.

General Indications and Applications

Experience with octyl-2-cyanoacrylate indicates its usefulness for closure of lacerations in the emergency room[7-10]; it reduces the amount of surgical time, causes less pain, and produces a satisfactory cosmetic result. It also is less traumatic for children in the treatment of lacerations of the face and scalp. When it is used in skin graft fixation along the margins, results obtained are comparable to those of sutures.[11] In neonates with prominent[11] aures, the glue has been applied in the mastoid region, establishing a scaffold for the cartilage growth. Although we do not yet have concrete data to present, our clinical experience indicates that this adhesive could offer a good alternative to the compressive nonsurgical method for treatment of prominent ears and to skin sutures in the repair of cleft lip[12] and in facelifts (especially in the periauricular area).

Other successful applications reported in the use of octyl-2-cyanoacrylate include the treatment of bleeding esophageal varices,[13] as an adhesive between the external ocular muscle of the ocular globe and an orbital implant.[14] It has also been used in the temporary treatment of facial paralysis[15] as an adhesive to stabilize external eyelid weight on the superior palpebra. These results opened many avenues for its application in surgical areas specific to plastic surgery.

Indications in Body Contouring

The octyl-2-cyanoacrylate (Dermabond) tissue glues have been used successfully in procedures such as mammaplasty, dermolipectomy, and abdominoplasty. It glues skin wound margins in a shorter time than traditional suture techniques. The results have been satisfactory with reduced operative time and cosmetic results similar to those achieved with sutures. It also has been cost-effective in closure of long wounds like abdominoplasty and body lifts as well as in incisions for breast augmentation and in closing wounds after the introduction of cannulas for liposuction. Its use in liposuction, however, is controversial, since drainage through this open wound is not possible when glue is applied (see box on p. 172).

Indications

Reduction mammaplasties	Gynecomastias
Augmentation mammaplasty	Liposuction (controversial)
Dermolipectomies	

Contraindications

Octyl-2-cyanoacrylate (Dermabond) should not be used on contaminated or infected wounds or on mucous membrane surfaces or mucocutaneous junctions, such as the lip and oral cavity. In our experience, adhesive polymer inside the wound produces an inflammatory reaction with formation of larger and wider scars. Its use also should be avoided in regions regularly exposed to fluids or in areas of dense hair such as the scalp. It should not be used in patients who are hypersensitive to cyanoacetate or formaldehyde. It also is not appropriate for closing wounds with excessive tension to avoid dehiscence over conventional suturing or over wet wounds, which can accelerate the process of polymerization.

Presentation and Preparation of Material

Octyl-2-cyanoacrylate (Dermabond) is available commerically in its monomeric liquid form combined with a violet dye. The monomer is contained in a sterile vial that measures 4.7 cm by 0.8 cm in diameter with a 0.5 ml volume.

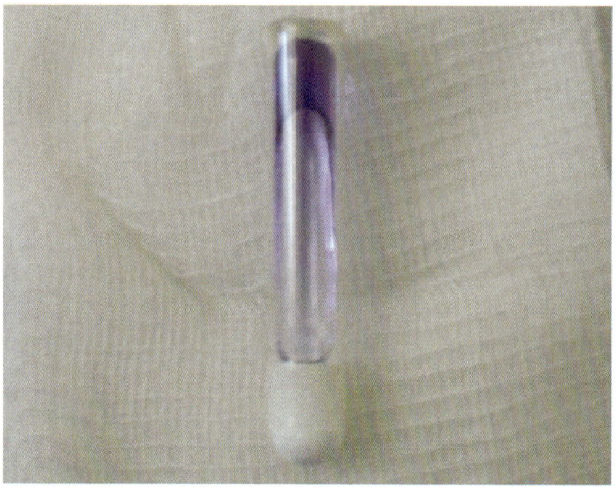

The vial has an internal glass breakable ampule that contains the monomer wrapped in a plastic shell connected to a semipermeable sponge applicator tip. The vial should be stored at temperatures below 30° C, protected from high humidity and light.

To activate the product, the ampule must be compressed firmly until the internal glass ampule ruptures. The monomer is expressed to the applicator tip with gentle digital compression. There is an initiator in the applicator tip that will accelerate polymerization as the adhesive is applied to the incision. It is important to emphasize that once started, the activation process is irreversible and the adhesive must be used immediately. Otherwise the product will polymerize while still inside the vial. Polymerization is accelerated when the monomer is exposed to moisture. Therefore, after contact with skin, the glue will polymerize within 20 to 50 seconds.

Application And Technique

The wound must be clean with no evidence of infection or foreign body with good hemostasis and no tension. Any tension at the margins of the incision should be minimized with absorbable dermal sutures (e.g., Vicryl, Monocryl, or PDS). We do not recommend the use of organic sutures like catgut because of the potential for local tissue reactions. The margins should be closely approximated to aid with the glue application.

After the dermal sutures have been placed, we recommend washing the wound with saline solution to remove any clots, fat, and so on. The wound margins are then dried and carefully prepared for perfect coaptation with skin edge eversion before the glue is applied. We believe that precise skin edge eversion is important because one may find it difficult to obtain good approximation of the wound margins as the glue is applied. Precise wound margin approximation can be accomplished using forceps or skin hooks and should be maintained for at least 10 to 30 seconds after the first pass of the glue applicator to insure proper position of the wound margins until the polymerization is complete. The manufacturer recommends the following steps to promote adequate skin closure:

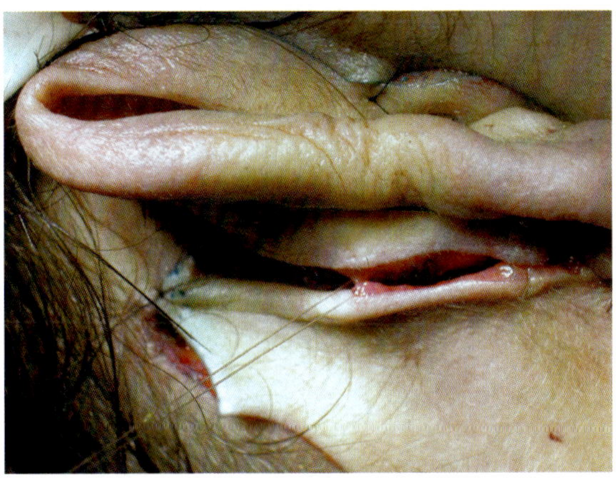

The wound is prepared with hemostasis and foreign body removal. Dermal sutures are placed at equivalent levels to eliminate subcutaneous dead space.

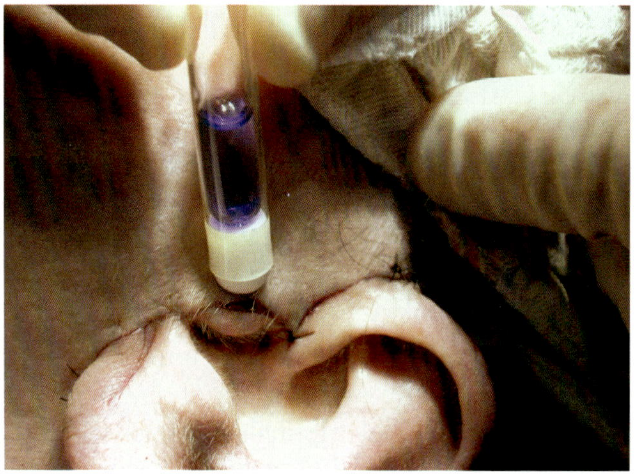

After the wound is cleaned, approximation of the wound margins is rehearsed and an effort is made to keep the skin edges everted. Hemostasis will need to be optimized because during the closure some blood may be expressed from the wound, which may prohibit adequate approximation of the skin edges.

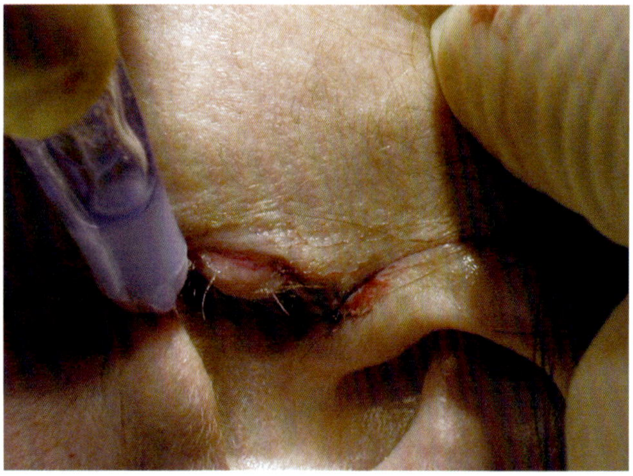

The internal glass ampule is ruptured by digital compression. The product is applied while keeping the margins approximated for 10 to 30 seconds to maintain good approximation of the wound margins during the polymerization process.

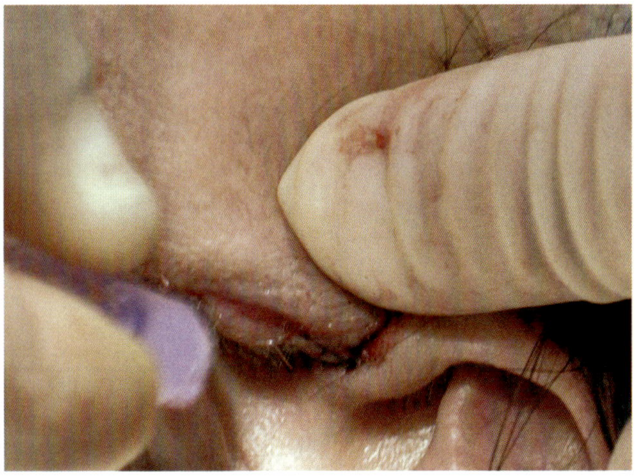

Two more passes are made with the applicator over 10 to 30 seconds.

Evaluation in Wound Care

Once the application is completed, there is no need for dressings. The wound is impermeable and the patient is free to shower. However, one should avoid immersion, bathing, and use of soap. The glue will start peeling off around 10 days following application of the cyanoacrylate.

Problems, Tricks, and Potential Complications

Some technical problems have been reported in the application of Dermabond when used improperly. One should avoid applying the glue inside the wound. This can cause a foreign body reaction with cyst formation, potential infection, and a possible delay in wound healing.[16] To avoid these problems, the skin edges must be kept closely approximated until the polymerization is completed during the first application. We recommend waiting 30 seconds while stabilizing the skin edges before more glue is applied. Another potential problem is the adhesion of other objects to the surgical wound (e.g., surgical gloves, dressings, etc.). This can be avoided by waiting 60 seconds before manipulating the polymer. Gauze can be used to remove the glue before it has fully polymerized.

When working around the eye, a potential complication is the inadvertent placement of the glue into the eye. Keeping the wound in a flat position will avoid running of the glue near important structures. Cyanoacrylates are less likely to adhere to an oily surface. By placing petroleum-based ointment around the periphery of the wound, one can minimize erroneous application. One should avoid excessive glue application as this can generate excessive heat of polymerization and the glue may remain in place for many weeks and require removal.

Case Examples

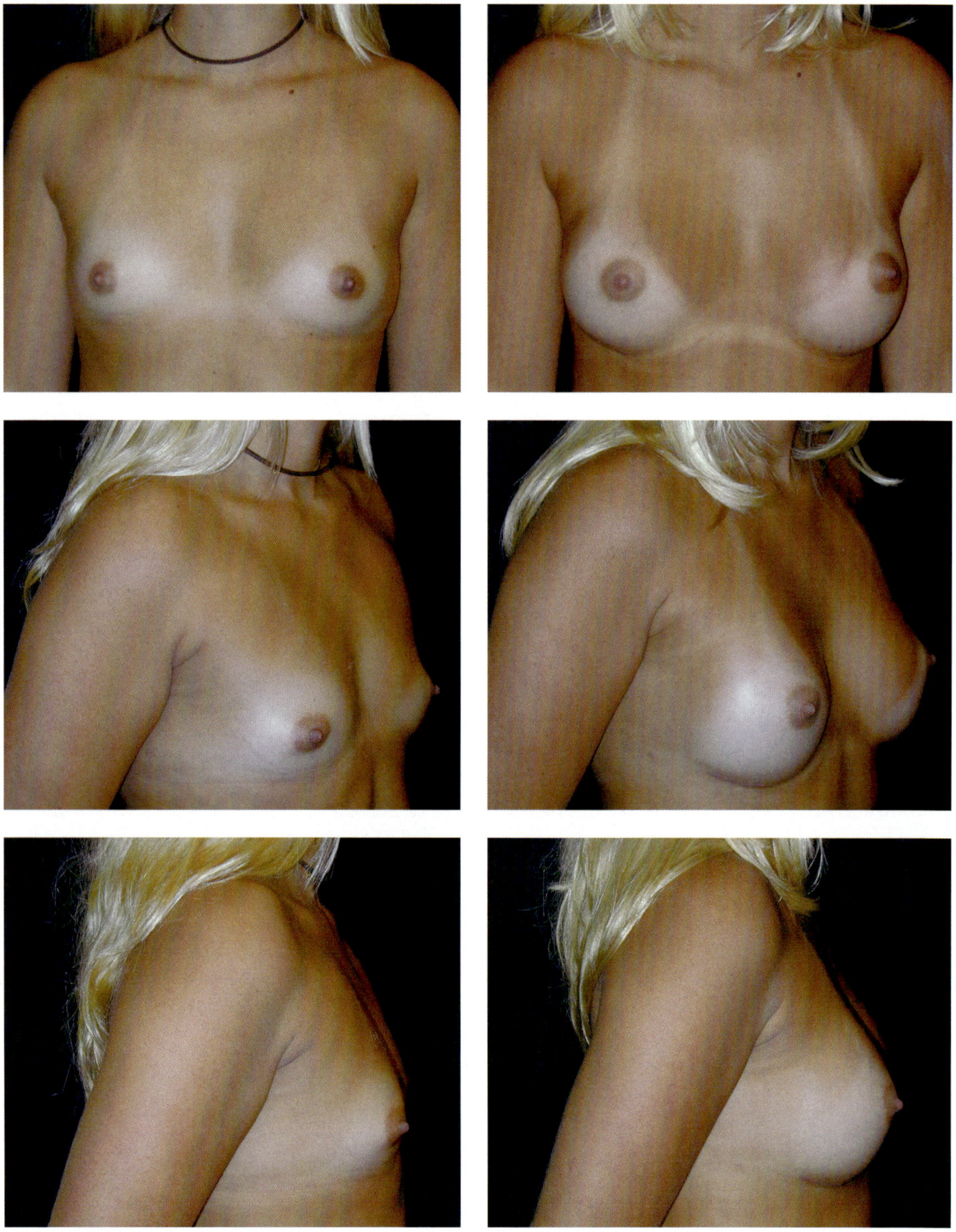

A 27-year-old white woman who underwent breast augmentation with retromuscular implants and inframammary incision. The wound was approximated with absorbable dermal sutures and Dermabond.

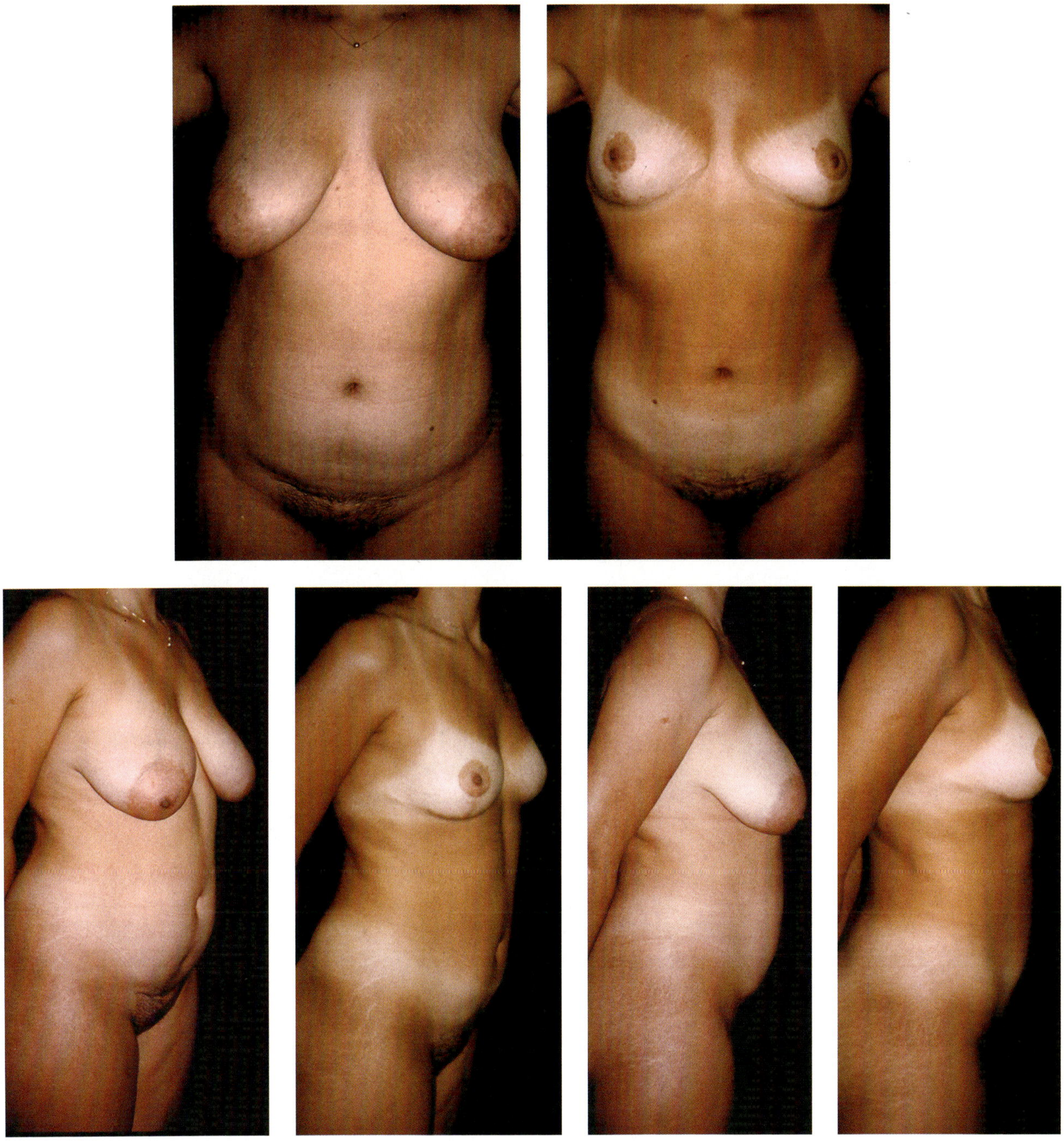

A 47-year-old woman who presented with a previous C-section scar and hypermastia. She underwent a reduction mammaplasty and abdominoplasty with revision of abdominal scar. All wounds were approximated with absorbable sutures and sealed with Dermabond.

Conclusion

Aesthetic results obtained with the use of octyl-2-cyanoacrylate appear to be similar to those obtained with traditional suture. There is also an appreciable reduction in surgical time with reduction of cost and complications. Patient comfort should not be underestimated. He or she is free to shower within hours after surgery because of the impermeable wound covering. The psychological advantage of no suture removal is clearly evident during the postoperative period especially in children.

We have observed excellent wound healing with the use of cyanoacrylate adhesives. The polymer also appears to promote compression at the wound margins during the maturation process and consequently reduces the collagen synthesis, generating an inconspicuous scar.

REFERENCES

1. Gosain AK, Lyon VB. The current status of tissue glues: Part II. For adhesion of soft tissue safety and efficacy report. Plastic Surgery Educational Foundation DATA Committee 110:1581-1584, 2002.
2. Trott AT. Cyanoacrylate tissue adhesives: An advance in wound care. JAMA 277:1559-1560, 1997.
3. Maw JL, Quinn JV, Wells GA, Ducic Y, Odell PF, Lamothe A, Brownrigg PJ, Sutcliffe T. A prospective comparison of octylcyanoacrylate tissue adhesive and suture for the closure of head and neck incisions. J Otolaryngol 26:26-30, 1997.
4. Ogus NT, Emir M, Çicek S, Isik O. Prevention of recurrent osteomyelitis using cyanoacrylate gluing in mediastinitis. Ann Thorac Surg 70:1761-1763, 2000.
5. Palmieri B. Attualità sui collanti biologici ad uso clinico: I cianoacrilati. Continental Medical Group Trieste, 1994.
6. Quinn J, Maw J, Ramotar K, Wenckebach G, Wells G. Octylcyanoacrylate tissue adhesive versus suture wound repair in a contaminated wound model. Surgery 122:69-72, 1997.
7. Farion K, Osmond MH, Hartling L, Russel K, Klassen T, Crumley E, Wiebe N. Tissue adhesives for traumatic lacerations in children and adults. Cochrane Database Syst Rev(3): CD003326, 2002.
8. Penoff J. Skin closures using cyanoacrylate tissue adhesives. Plast Reconstr Surg 103:730-731, 1999.
9. Bernard L, Doyle J, Friedlander SF, Eichenfield LF, Gibbs NF, Cunningham BB. A prospective comparison of octyl cyanoacrylate tissue adhesive (Dermabond) and suture for the closure of excisional wounds in children and adolescents. Arch Dermatol 137:1177-1180, 2001.
10. Bruns T, Robinson BS, Smith RJ, Kile DL, Davis TP, Sullivan KM, Quinn JV. A new tissue adhesive for laceration repair in children. J Pediatr 132:1067-1070, 1998.
11. Hallock GG. Expanded applications for octyl-2-cyanoacrylate as a tissue adhesive. Ann Plast Surg 46:185-189, 2001.
12. Magee WP, Ajkay N, Githae B, Rosenblun RS. Use of octyl-2-cyanoacrylate in cleft lip repair. Ann Plast Surg 50:1-5, 2003.
13. Nguyen AJ, Baron TH, Burgart LJ, Leontovich O, Rajan E, Gostout CJ. 2-Octyl-cyanoacrylate (Dermabond), a new glue for variceal injection therapy: Results of a preliminary animal study. Gastrointest Endosc 55:572-575, 2002.

14. Gupta BK, Edward D, Duffy MT. 2-Octyl cyanoacrilate tissue adhesive and muscle attachment to porous anophtalmic orbital implants. Ophthal Plast Reconstr Surg 17:264-269, 2001.
15. Shepler TR, Seiff SR. Use of isobutyl cyanoacrylate tissue adhesive to stabilize external eyelid weights in temporary treatment of facial palsies. Ophthal Plast Reconstr Surg 17: 169-173, 2001.
16. Toriumi DM, Raslan WF, Friedman M, Tardy ME Jr. Variable histotoxicity of Histoacryl when used in a subcutaneous site: An experimental study. Laryngoscope 101:339-343, 1991.

CHAPTER

11

Tissue Adhesives: Current Status and Future Directions

Ian T. Jackson, M.D., D.Sc.(Hon.) ▪
Barbara J. Beal, B.S., R.N. ▪ Christopher P. Kelly, M.D. ▪
Renato Saltz, M.D.

Tissue adhesives have become an integral part of plastic surgery practice today. While there are multiple applications for these products, they are primarily used for suture support, tissue adhesion, and hemostasis. It is this last use that makes tissue adhesives effective and highly useful in surgery. Tissue sealing is imperative to wound healing, and the use of tissue adhesives offers significant advantages in terms of decreased morbidity, excellent cosmesis, and reduced costs.

Fibrin glues are the most widely used tissue adhesives in surgery, because they are safe and promote healing. Other adhesives, including cyanoacrylates, albumin-based compounds, collagen-based compounds, glutaraldehyde glues, and hydrogels,[1] also offer significant promise.

Available Products and Current Applications

Fibrin Glues

Fibrin glues are either autologous or commercially prepared. For preparation of autologous fibrin glue, 50 ml of the patient's blood is collected in a citrated tube. The plasma supernatant, which contains fibrinogen, is removed by plasmapheresis. Plasma is then added to a solution of thrombin and calcium to form fibrin on the wound bed. Studies have shown that increasing the fibrinogen concentration of the glue increases its adhesive strength.[2] Fibrinogen concentration can be increased either by concentrating the fibrinogen taken from a single donor or pooling the fibrinogen obtained from multiple donors.

Commercially prepared fibrin glues are used extensively in Europe, Canada, and Japan, but only two have been approved by the Food and Drug Administration (FDA) for use in the United States (Tisseel, Baxter Corporation, Deerfield, Ill.; and Hemaseel APR, Haemacure Corporation, Montreal, Quebec, Canada). These products undergo donor screening, heat treating, and the use of a solvent detergent suspension to inactivate lipid-enveloped bloodborne viruses to make them safer. Obviously, single-donor or autologous products increase the safety margin. Most commercial pooled fibrin glue products and products derived from autologous fibrinogen contain thrombin, which activates the fibrinogen.[2] Human thrombin preparations are used rather than bovine thrombin because several cases of anaphylaxis were reported along with antibody formation to bovine factor V, which depleted human factor V in several patients.[3]

In the commercially prepared fibrin sealant, a solution of fibrinogen in cryoprecipitate is mixed with a solution of thrombin and applied to the bleeding site. Hemostasis is achieved in 3 to 5 seconds.[4] The fibrin glue forms a strong bond that interacts with the molecular structure of the damaged tissue and begins to mimic the final stage of the coagulation cascade. Staindl[5] reported that the application of split-thickness and full-thickness skin grafts with fibrin glue to wounds of the nose, ear, and face "exhibited atraumatic and stronger fixation effects than those of conventional suture fixation."

Fibrin glues are simple to use, inexpensive, and safe. They are bioabsorbable and biodegradable. Because of their excellent safety record in the United States and Europe, fibrin glues are used extensively in many surgical specialties. There have been numerous articles written on the clinical uses of fibrin glue.[2,6-9] What makes them so attractive for use in plastic surgery is the potential economic impact and positive outcome for these patients.

The advantages of fibrin glues in plastic and reconstructive surgery can be summarized as follows:

- Significant reduction of hematomas
- Sealing of tissues
- Less suturing
- Decrease in postoperative healing time

Cyanoacrylates

Cyanoacrylates were first used during the Vietnam era to help with wound closures. Although these tissue adhesives are stronger than fibrin sealants, their use is more limited. Their primary application is for skin reapproximation. Cyanoacrylates are foreign bodies that could induce internal inflammation, tissue necrosis, and infection risks[10]; consequently they are recommended only for topical use.[11]

Dermabond (Ethicon, Somerville, N.J.) is a 2-octyl cyanoacrylate and has been approved for use in the United States.[12] It is used in emergency rooms to close smaller cuts or to reapproximate lacerations for which deeper sutures have been used for support. Plastic surgeons use it in areas where skin sutures are avoided for cosmetic reasons. Because Dermabond is waterproof, a dressing is unnecessary. It is helpful for treating small cuts in children who are afraid of needles. It is effective for 7 to 10 days, but its use should be limited to the repair of small wounds and lacerations.[1] Dermabond has been prospectively compared with suture closure for skin lacerations of the head and neck, and no differences were noted cosmetically; however, these were scored from photographs taken up to 12 weeks postoperatively.

Albumin-Based Compounds (Glutaraldehyde Glues)

This group of adhesives is a combination of albumin and adhesion compounds. They are referred to as *gelatin-resorcinol-formaldehyde glutaraldehyde (GRFG) glues.* There is one compound approved in the United States for limited use in the repair of aortic dissection.[1] This product combines bovine albumin and glutaraldehyde glue and is known as BioGlue (CryoLife, Inc., Kennesaw, Ga.). It has been approved for use in surgical repair of acute thoracic aortic dissection. This adhesive is based on a combination of albumin and adhesion compounds; it polymerizes immediately and forms a firm adhesive bond.[13] Pending further studies, BioGlue appears to be an effective tissue glue. It is composed of bovine albumin and glutaraldehyde glue and is related to the GRFG glues used in other countries for vascular and pulmonary procedures. An important aspect of BioGlue is that the formaldehyde component is taken out because of its toxic properties. BioGlue fills in the dissection, thereby closing the cavity and providing a stronger arterial wall for the repair. It has a half-life of approximately 30 days. FDA approval for BioGlue is limited because long-term outcomes are not yet known.[14]

Hydrogels

Polyethylene glycol (PEG) polymers are hydrogels developed for tissue adhesion. PEG, a water-soluble agent activated by light, was developed by Genzyme Biosurgery (Cambridge, Mass.). The product's name is FocalSeal-L; it is applied to tissue and used with a light source to activate its adhesion. It takes time to apply and set, but it is bioabsorbable and biodegradable (it biodegrades in 3 months). A disadvantage is that FocalSeal-L is difficult to apply, especially when bleeding is profuse.[1] FocalSeal-L has helped to decrease the incidence of air leaks after major thoracic surgery. Although it has been approved by the FDA, its role in medicine is not yet established.[13]

Collagen-Based Adhesive

Collagen-based adhesive is relatively new. It is exciting because it works by providing a matrix for the clot and aids coagulation by delivering fibrinogen to the area. This adhesive has been approved for use in the United States under the brand name FloSeal (Baxter Corporation, Deerfield, Ill.). It is made from a combination of bovine collagen and bovine thrombin. FloSeal is widely used in ear, nose, and throat surgery (e.g., endoscopic sinus surgery), in vascular surgery for hemostasis,[15] in plastic surgery for high-flow vascular lesions, and recently in aesthetic surgery for rhytidectomies. It is also used in neurosurgery for the treatment of cerebrospinal fluid leaks.[16] In our experience, this adhesive has been very useful for the severe bleeding encountered in excision of head and neck tumors and for troublesome bleeding during facelifts.

Clinical Applications

Tissue Glues in Aesthetic Surgery

Clinical and Laboratory Studies

Clinical and laboratory studies in the literature lend validity to the benefits derived from the use of tissue glues in aesthetic surgery. Fezza et al.[8] used aerosolized fibrin glue in 24 of 48 facelifts. The group on whom he used fibrin glue clinically had less bruising, less edema, and a faster healing response. Fewer hematomas formed and, more significantly, no drains were used.

Marchac and Sandor[9] did an analysis of 200 patients who had facelifts and reported similar results, few complications, improved healing, and possibly less extensive surgery when glue is used. According to Fezza et al.,[8] the operating time for facelifts decreased by 13.3 minutes because less time was required for cauterizing as the surgeon became confident of the capabilities of tissue glue. Drains were not used, thus decreasing the operating time. In blepharoplasty and when sprayed on newly resurfaced skin, aerosolized fibrin glue is especially promising and convenient to use.

In a study conducted by Grossman et al.,[17] the complications of seroma and skin necrosis were tied to problems of failure of the glue to dissolve properly during preparation, improper patient positioning, and inconsistent application of the sealant, along with timing of the application. The benefits of using fibrin glue included hemostasis, closer approximation of tissues, less postoperative edema, and ecchymosis.[17] Studies by Bruck[7] showed fibrin glue to be efficacious in controlling slow bleeding foci, diffuse oozing, and lymphatic leaks. He initially used a two-component tissue adhesive, the sealant-concentrated fibrinogen—factor XIII and "other proteins"—and a "hardener," thrombin and calcium chloride. This produced a rigid clot. The addition of aprotinin, a fibrinolysis inhibitor, controls decay of the newly formed fibrinogen. In a series of 82 consecutive facelifts, the skin was glued down well, and preauricular sutures were unnecessary. Patients had diminished postoperative swelling and no complications.[7] Staindl[5] reported the efficacy of fibrin glue with improved hemostasis in head and neck surgery. Grossman et al.[17] used fibrin sealant in 105 patients who underwent 128 facial aesthetic procedures, including facelifts, coronal browlifts, temporal tucks, midface rejuvenations, and neck lifts, and reported excellent results.

Clinical Experience
Tissue Glues in Aesthetic Surgery
Renato Saltz

The trend in aesthetic surgery practices today is to offer patients a total package of treatments, with an emphasis on antiaging and therapies that contribute to the patient's total health, rejuvenation, and fitness. Consequently the modern plastic surgery practice will offer a range of services. Surgical procedures such as liposuction and body contouring, rhytidectomy, blepharoplasty, browlift, and rhinoplasty remain standard to most cosmetic surgery practices and a mainstay of what aesthetic surgeons do. Increasingly, however, skin care, tissue fillers (e.g., fat, Botox, Restalyn, and collagen), microdermabrasion, lasers, facials, makeup consultations, and even spa services and lymphatic drainage massage are being incorporated into this total aesthetic treatment plan to offer patients the comprehensive care they are requesting. Lymphatic drainage massage provides a means to reduce swelling, decrease discomfort, and improve patient satisfaction in the early postoperative period after facial rejuvenation or body contouring. The trend is for outpatient procedures, with less morbidity and a rapid recovery. Tissue glues are a natural component of this equation. They are particularly appealing when combined with endoscopic techniques, where the emphasis is on shorter scars with less morbidity. Tissue sealants enhance the results of minimally invasive surgery by reducing the rate of complications and other surgical sequelae, such as hematoma, seroma, bruising, and swelling. Plastic surgeons have readily incorporated tissue sealants in minimally invasive facial rejuvenation surgery, and these adhesives contribute to hemostasis and patient comfort because the need for drains is eliminated.

Fibrin-based sealants are potent hemostatic agents, sealants, and adhesives. Different applicators have been developed to deliver these sealants endoscopically, including spray systems and double syringes for more localized and superficial use (Figs. 11-1 through 11-3). Fibrin products are applied directly under the skin but directly over the soft tissues. One of the keys to a successful outcome when using tissue glues appears to be in the preparation and application of the fibrin sealant.[17] Aerosolized fibrin glue offers advantages in aesthetic surgery because less glue is wasted and a fine mist delivers the glue evenly to avoid "clumping," which could impede healing.

The major nonfibrin sealant is Dermabond, a modified cyanoacrylate based in a liquid adhesive that has been available in the United States since 1998 (see p. 183 for further discussion). It glues skin wound margins in a shorter time than with traditional suturing techniques. It has been shown to be cost-effective in closure of long wounds such as abdominoplasty, breast surgery, and body lifts and can act as an antimicrobial barrier with possible infection reduction in the immediate postoperative period. It also avoids suture removal in the postoperative period causing patients less discomfort and creating increased patient satisfaction.

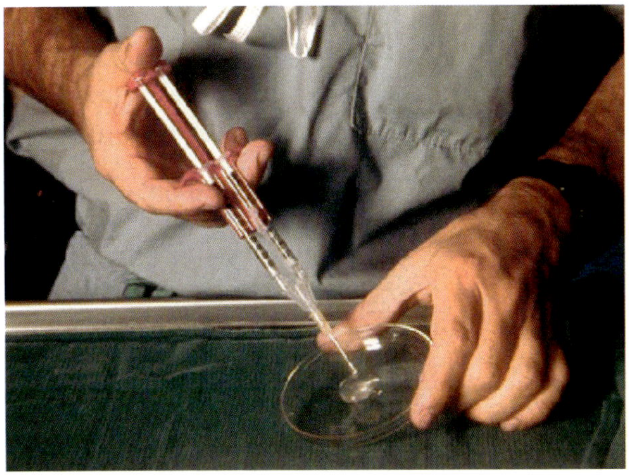

Figure 11-1 Dual-syringe applicator of fibrin sealant.

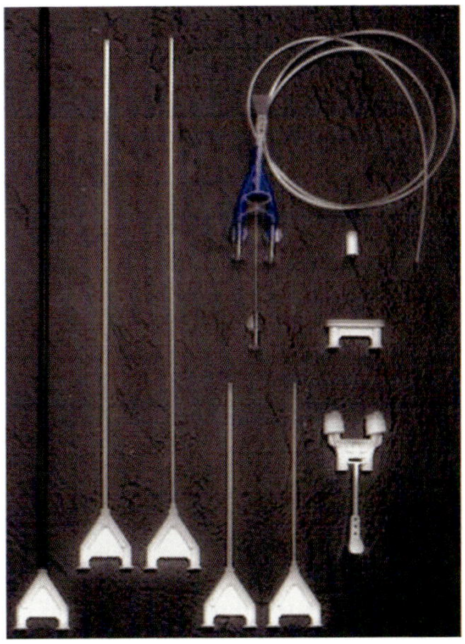

Figure 11-2 Endoscopic applicators of fibrin sealant.

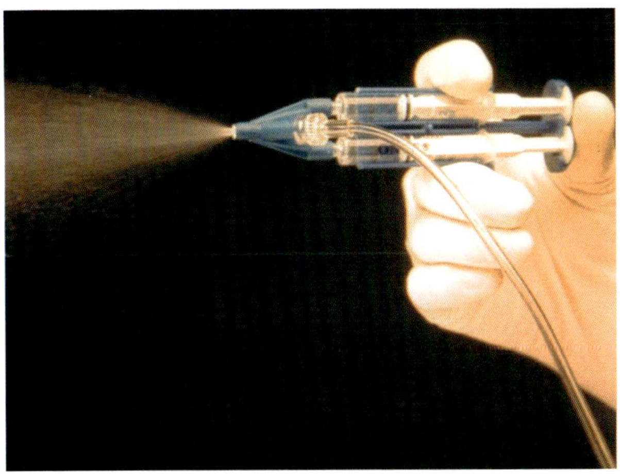

Figure 11-3 Spray applicator of fibrin sealant.

Tissue glues have been used in endoscopic browlift and midface suspension since the mid-1990s. The endoscopic approach has been well described and consists of the following three stages: (1) subperiosteal undermining and dissection in the temporal area over the deep temporal fascia, communicating with extensive subperiosteal undermining over the frontal bone; (2) periosteal release, including the retaining ligament junction of the deep temporal fascia and periosteum; and (3) fixation of soft tissues. Endoscopic undermining along the lateral orbital rim allows the surgeon to access the midface and through careful, magnified endoscopic dissection, visualize and preserve important vascular and neurosensory structures.

Over the past 10 years the need for fixation—and the best type of fixation—in endoscopic browlift and midface suspension have been widely debated. Once a complete release of the supraorbital periosteum is complete, some fixation method is indicated. In my experience, fibrin glue provides an excellent adhesive. In young patients with no significant brow ptosis, I have applied only fibrin glue with considerable success. In cases in which the midface has also been undermined and suspended using direct needle fixation technique, fibrin adhesive has helped to glue the soft tissues, minimize bleeding, seal the lymphatic channels, reduce lymphatic drainage, and decrease postoperative swelling and the incidence of seroma and hematoma.[37] In these cases I prefer to use the long endoscopic applicator for the midface and the double syringe for the temporal and frontal areas (Fig. 11-4). In my experience, tissue glues help eyebrow fixation by minimizing formation of small hematomas and seromas in the forehead and promoting better adhesion of the periosteum to the frontal bone as well as in the temporal region by allowing better sealing and adhesion.

During rhytidectomy, the superficial musculoaponeurotic system placation and platysmal plication are done first, then the preauricular and postauricular skin margins are trimmed prior to glue application to avoid manipulation of the skin flap after spraying. Hemostasis must be established before application of the fibrin sealant. The sealant is applied in the entire region with a spray system (Fig. 11-5), and soft pressure is applied for approximately 5 minutes. The side of the face is protected, the head is turned, and the same technique is used on the other side. Deep dermal absorbable sutures approximate the wound margins of preauricular and postauricular incisions, which are then sealed with Dermabond. The wound margins need to be completely dry and are approximated with nontension sutures. I always defat the preauricular tissue to recreate the pretragal sulcus and improve the aesthetic final appearance of the preauricular scar (Fig. 11-6).

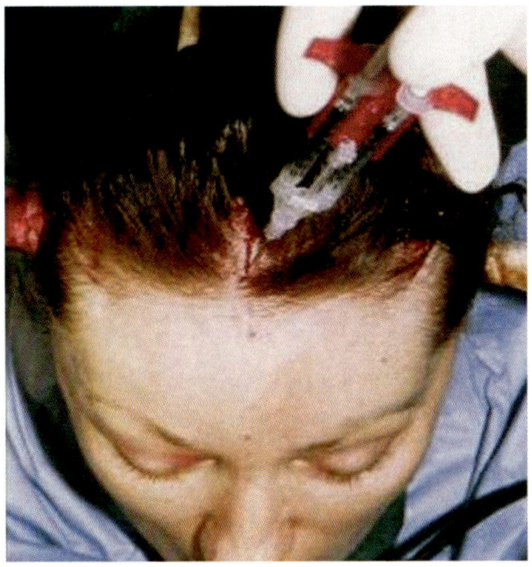

Figure 11-4 Application of tissue glues in endoscopic browlift.

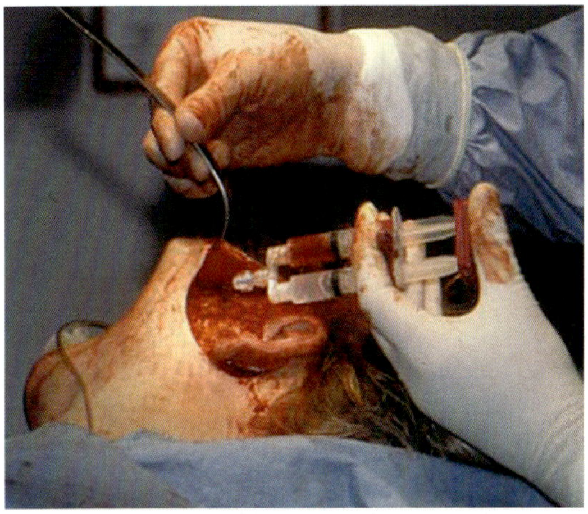

Figure 11-5 Spray system used during rhytidectomy.

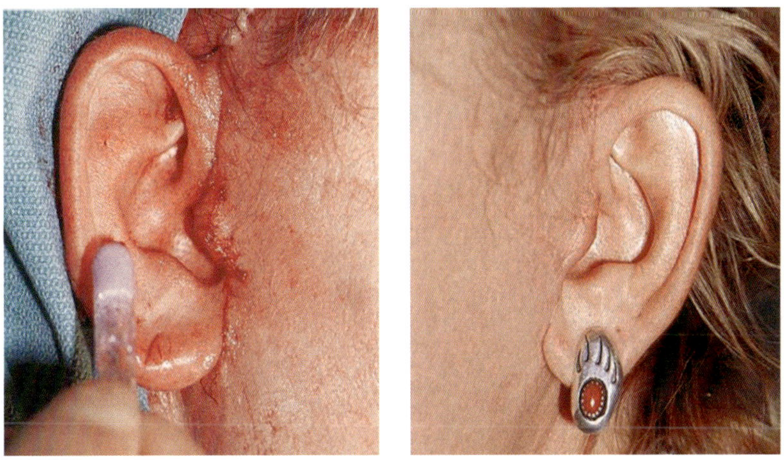

A

B

Figure 11-6 **A,** Tension-free skin approximation with dermal sutures and preauricular wound closure with Dermabond. **B,** Excellent aesthetic result at 6 months.

The same technique is applied to the submental wound. Face and hair are washed and shampooed before the patient is moved to the recovery room. The patient usually spends the night in the surgery center and is discharged the next morning (Figs. 11-7 through 11-10).

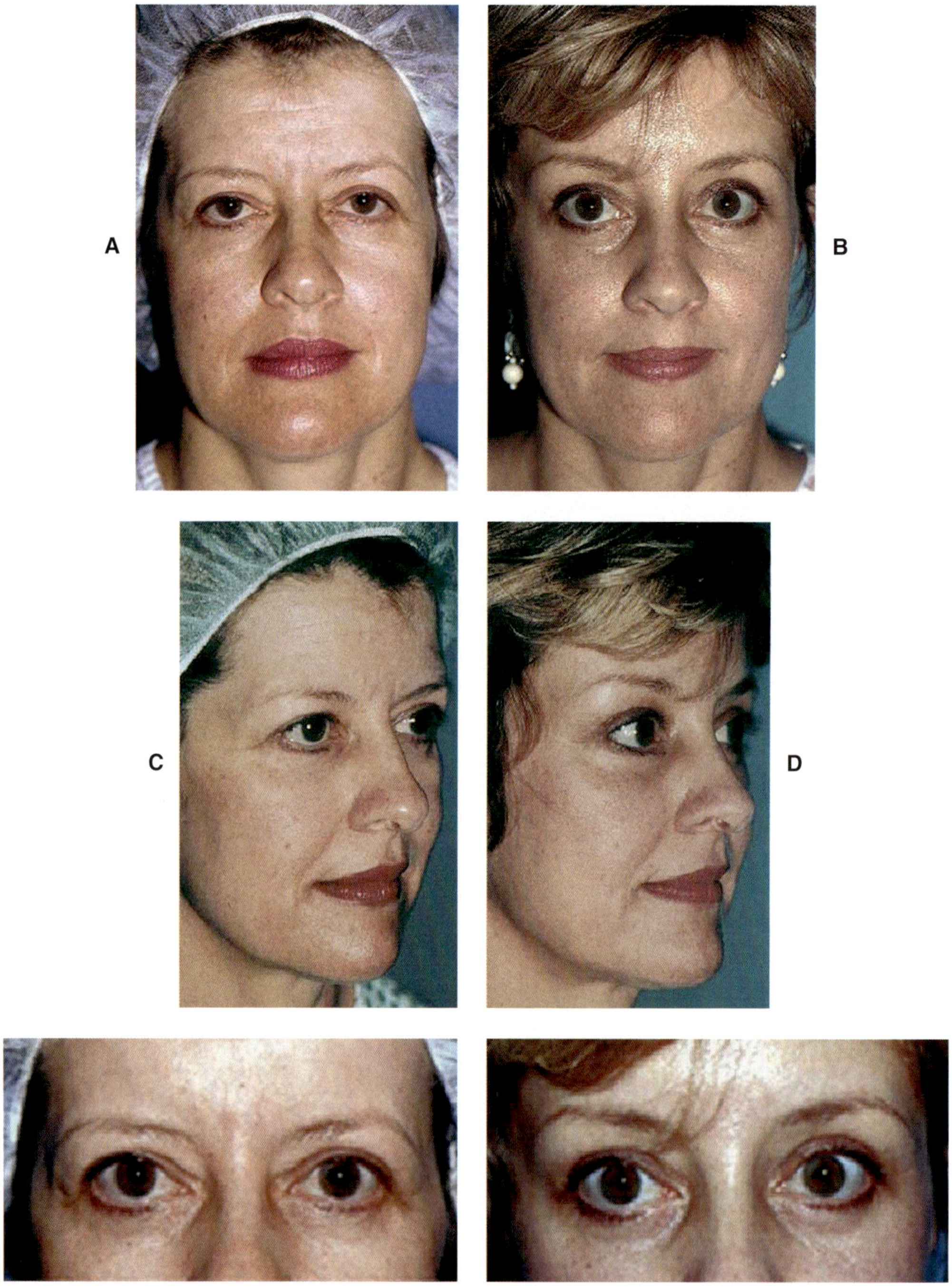

Figure 11-7 One-year results of endobrow fixation with tissue glues. **A** and **B,** Front view. **C** and **D,** Oblique view. **E** and **F,** Browlift as treatment for temporal hooding and mild brow ptosis. Fixation was done with tissue sealant.

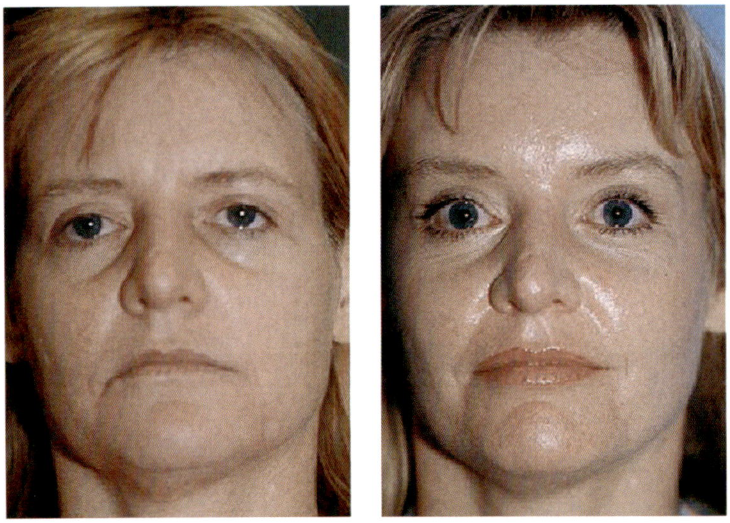

Figure 11-8 Endoscopic browlift and midface suspension with direct needle fixation. Tissue sealant was applied to the forehead and midface.

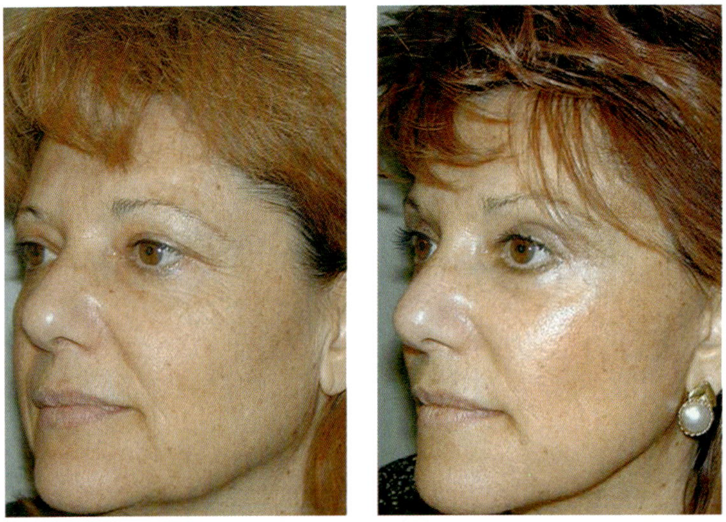

Figure 11-9 Endoscopic browlift with rhytidectomy and cervicoplasty. Tissue sealants were applied to the forehead, face, and neck. Dermabond was applied to seal preauricular and submental incisions.

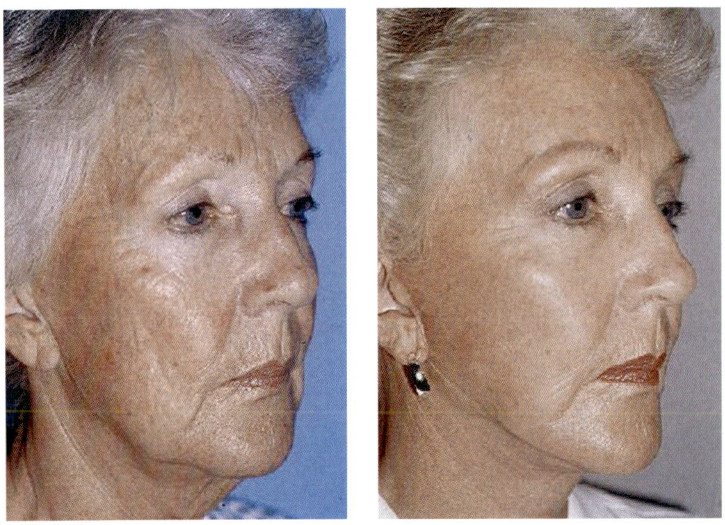

Figure 11-10 Secondary endoscopic browlift with rhytidectomy and cervicoplasty. Tissue sealants were applied to the forehead, face, and neck. Dermabond was applied to seal preauricular and submental incisions.

When fibrin glue is applied with the Duploject syringe, caution must be exercised to avoid depositing a large amount of glue in one small area, which could serve as a barrier to revascularization and by compression cause localized ischemia, resulting in tissue necrosis.

The use of tissue sealants has significantly decreased the use of drains and dressings in facial rejuvenation surgery in my practice. On postoperative day 2, the patient returns to the clinic and is started on lymphatic drainage massage by a certified medical massage therapist. The patient learns the advantages of these early interventional techniques and starts using them at home as early as the first postoperative week. Because all of the exposed scars have been sealed with Dermabond, they have been washed and cared for since the recovery room. During the first postoperative clinic visit, the patient is seen by a makeup artist who helps to apply postoperative camouflage makeup to cover fresh scars and bruises (Fig. 11-11).

I have used tissue glues and sealants for facial rejuvenation surgery since 1987. Dermabond has been added more recently to these procedures. The addition of massage with instruction in camouflage makeup in the early postoperative period has completed and redefined the concept of minimally invasive facial rejuvenation in my practice. Patients feel well in the early postoperative period and are able to return to work within days with a remarkable decrease in swelling, bruising, and ecchymosis. This approach also adds to patient satisfaction and tends to reduce or avoid the mild postoperative depression commonly seen after facelift surgery (Fig. 11-12).

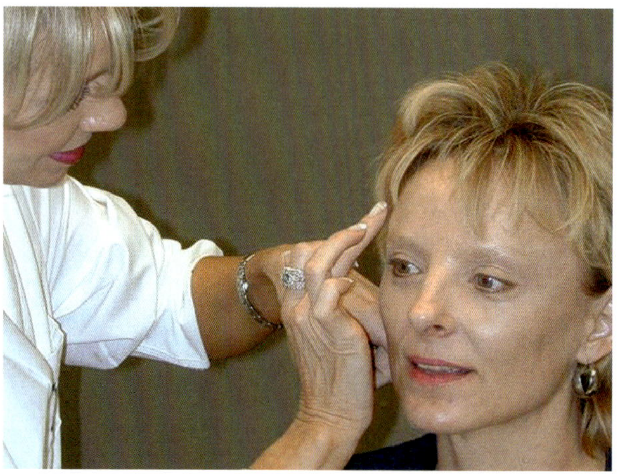

Figure 11-11 Patient is shown 7 days after endoscopic browlift and midface suspension with direct needle fixation. Tissue sealants were applied to forehead and midface areas. Minimal swelling and bruising is observed permitting an earlier return to work and greater patient satisfaction.

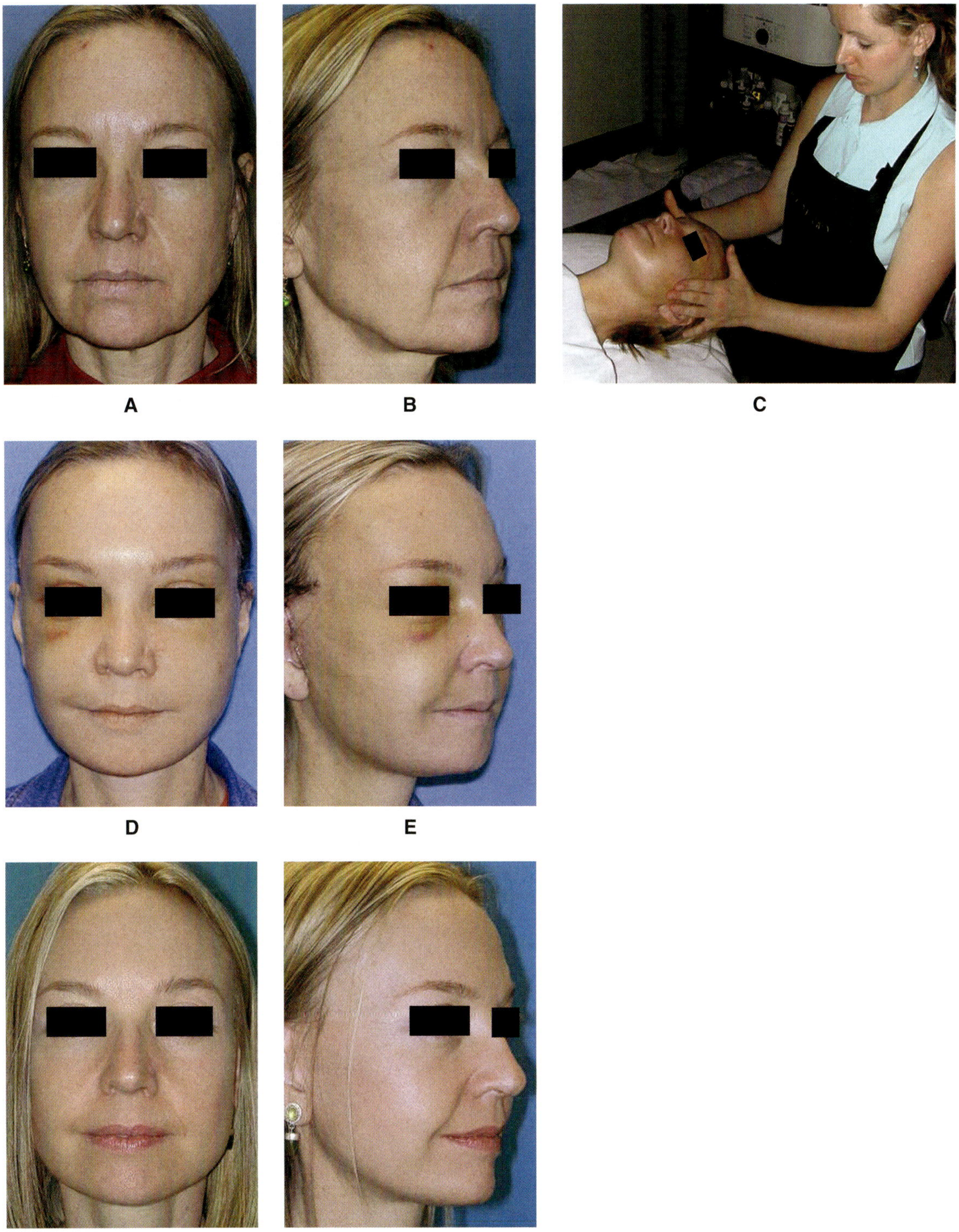

A B C D E F G

Figure 11-12 A and **B,** Patient candidate for facial rejuvenation surgery. **C,** Lymphatic drainage massage was performed on postoperative day 2. **D** and **E,** Day 4 following endoscopic browlift, midface suspension, rhytidectomy, and cervicoplasty. Tissue sealants and early lymphatic drainage massage decrease bruising and swelling, reducing patient discomfort and increasing patient satisfaction. **F** and **G,** Results at 4 months.

Tissue Glues in Reconstructive Surgery

Clinical and Laboratory Studies

The effects of fibrin glues have been studied extensively in the treatment of burn wounds. Vibe and Pless[18] of Denmark, in 1983, compared the use of Tisseel with catgut suturing with bolsters for stabilizing skin grafts. At 10 days, the Tisseel-stabilized grafts showed only a slightly better take (92% vs. 83%) in difficult areas, such as the neck and the scapula. The graft take with Tisseel was better (88% vs. 44%).

In another study, four different groups of patients, facial burns, hand burns, difficult graft sites, and miscellaneous surgical applications had either autologous or single-donor fibrin glue in which Saltz et al.[6] obtained better functional and cosmetic results with decreased blood loss and enhanced graft survival.

Greenhalgh et al.[19] observed that when autologous fibrin glue was used, the graft sites treated with fibrin appeared to accelerate the maturation of burn-related scarring; graft sites appeared to lose their reddened appearance by 7 to 8 months (usually it is expected that it will take 9 to 12 months for this to happen). Greenhalgh advised that additional investigations are needed to determine whether a component of human fibrin sealant accelerates the maturation phase of tissue repair. Fibrin glues have also been used successfully to improve skin graft survival, especially in areas where grafts are difficult to immobilize. Adant et al.[20] used fibrin glue on split-thickness skin grafts and demonstrated better adhesive take and improved cosmetic results.

Chakravorty and Sosnowski[21] also demonstrated similar results with full-thickness skin grafts. Grafts treated with fibrin sealant contracted significantly less than control grafts from postgraft day 9 until the end of the study. Gosain and Lyon[22] reported a reduction in bacteria in the recipient bed because bacteria grow slower in a clot of fibrinogen glue than in a physiologic clot. There is also evidence that fibrin glue aids in wound healing with increased angiogenesis and fibroblast ingrowth seen in the wound bed.

Fibrin glues have been used to aid in wound healing and provide tissue sealing where sutures cannot control bleeding or may stimulate it. According to Spotnitz et al.,[23] their ability as a suture support may eventually decrease the amount of sutures needed and may lead to an improved cosmetic result. Vibe and Pless[18] demonstrated a significant advantage in applying the fibrin adhesive to difficult recipient sites. Ihara et al.[24] showed that the hemostatic effect in fixation of skin grafts was augmented with the use of fibrin glue. They also documented fewer blood transfusions, shorter operative time, and reduced lengths of stay in the hospital for those patients. Stuart et al.[25] confirmed some of these results.

Although adhesion formation may occur with the use of fibrin glue, no articles have been published that confirm this.[26] However, numerous investigators have found fibrin glue to be effective in controlling adhesions.[27-30]

Fibrin glues have proved their efficacy in the surgical setting. In addition to closure of skin, fibrin glues are the best choice for hemostasis and wound sealing. They have been used successfully to seal dural leaks, lymphocytes, and on the dura to control cerebrospinal fluid leaks. Fibrin glues have also been shown to aid wound healing. Saltz et al.[6] cited studies reporting almost invisible scarring when fibrin glue was used on skin healing or on parenchymal injuries in rabbits.

Fibrin sealants are also effective in the prevention of seromas. Seromas are difficult problems to treat and can lead to infection, wound dehiscence, and tissue necrosis. Kulber et al.[31] used fibrin glue after harvesting the latissimus dorsi muscle in rats and found improved wound healing clinically with less skin flap necrosis. Fibrin sealant is ideal for preventing seromas because it acts as an adhesive that eliminates dead space, "seals tissue channels and facilities wound healing." A limitation of fibrin glue is its decreased adhesive properties when used in areas prone to fluid leakage.[32] Fibrin glue can be very useful for the treatment of recurrent seroma after abdominoplasty that has failed to subside after repeated needle aspirations (Fig. 11-13).

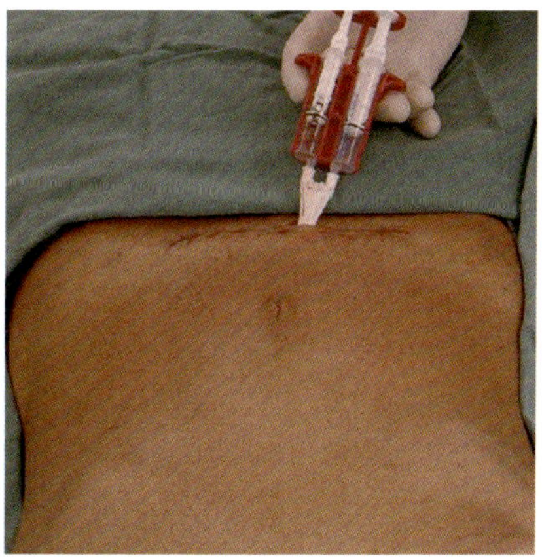

Figure 11-13 Recurrent seroma after abdominoplasty. The seroma capsule is "roughened" with a liposuction cannula (suction off) and then tissue sealant is applied with a dual syringe and a long catheter applicator. Compression and avoidance of exercise follow.

Clinical Experience With Patients With Burns

Renato Saltz

Surgical excision and immediate grafting in the early period after burn injury has gained increasing acceptance in the management of burns to the face and hands. There are several distinct advantages to the use of fibrin adhesive: (1) the autologous technique eliminates the risk of transmissible viral diseases (e.g., AIDS, hepatitis); (2) it can be used as a sealant in the treatment of seromas, dural leaks, and lymphoceles; and (3) it improves hemostasis and early graft adherence. Face and hands are resurfaced with sheet grafts in a single procedure, obtaining a better aesthetic result with complete graft take so that physical therapy can be initiated immediately. Other advantages include a decrease in the total number of anesthetics needed and a decrease in convalescence time.[11,12] Patients are able to move, eat, and ambulate on postoperative day 1. Color and texture matches have been very satisfactory in treated patients who now have been followed for more than a year. Neither sutures nor pressure dressings are required. There is minimal postoperative care and an early return to normal activities, which seems to increase the satisfaction of patients and nursing personnel.

In our experience, the usual resurfacing of facial burns with sheet grafts still demands significant, prolonged postoperative care and often results in a suboptimal graft take. In an attempt to obtain better function and appearance, minimal blood loss, and increased graft survival with minimal postoperative care, we decided to treat deep facial burns by sequential excision and grafting and to secure the grafts with autologous fibrin glue in one single operation.

In a retrospective, noncontrolled review of our experience with autologous fibrin glue in the treatment of facial burns and burns at difficult sites over a 14-month period, the beneficial effects of fibrin glue for burn patients was underscored.[33] A marked improvement in hemostasis and graft adherence combined with an excellent rate of graft take was observed in two clinical series. The use of autologous fibrin glue did not appear to increase the incidence of wound infection. Autologous fibrin glue eliminated the risk of transmission of viral disease. Clinical observation revealed that pressure dressings are not necessary and that minimal postoperative care was required; some burn patients can even be treated as outpatients.

In another study conducted from December 1987 to January 1990, 73 patients benefited from the use of autologous and single-donor fibrin glue.[34] Fifty-one wounds resulted from burns and 31 from other injuries, for a total of 82 applications. Facial burns in 19 patients were resurfaced in a single procedure with the help of fibrin glue. In four patients the entire face was reconstructed with aesthetic units. Facial burns that were not healed in 10 days were tangentially excised down to viable tissue and immediately grafted with medium-thickness skin sheet grafts. All grafts were secured in place with autologous or single-donor fibrin adhesive in accordance with the aesthetic units of the face. The grafts were obtained from the most suitable donor site with an appropriate match in color and skin texture. Gentle, uniform pressure was applied over the entire unit for 2 to 3 minutes immediately after the glue was applied. A few absorbable sutures were placed at the corners of the mouth and eyes, permitting early feeding and motion. After graft application, Xeroform dressing was placed over the entire unit. Eleven patients with deep second- or third-degree hand burns underwent early excision and grafting. Sheet grafts secured with autologous or single-donor fibrin glues were used to resurface the burn wound. These patients were intravenously resuscitated and treated with Silvadene dressings for 26 to 48 hours. After an accurate estimate of burn depth, definitive surgical care was begun. A total of 19 hands were treated in this group.

Fibrin glue was used to improve the early adherence of skin grafts in 32 difficult wounds that otherwise would have required bolster-type dressings and long-term immobilization. These areas included burns to the scalp (1), neck (9), extremities (2), trunk (3), and genitals (4) resulting from excision of hidradenitis suppurativa and Fournier's disease. They also included coverage of leg ulcers caused by venous stasis disease and vasculitis (5), various areas with great mobility where previously attempted skin grafting failed (2), and resurfacing of the forearm (4).

Fifteen patients had facial burns in which isolated aesthetic units were replaced. Four required the use of single-donor fibrin glue because of the magnitude of their burns and because they had previously received blood transfusions. The other 11 also benefited from the use of autologous fibrin glue.

The advantages of tangential excision and immediate grafting after burn injuries include shorter periods of hospitalization and a decreased number of operative procedures.[35,36] Despite these benefits, problems remain with current technique, including poor aesthetic results, hypertrophic scars, graft loss, blood loss, and other issues. We have obtained better functional and cosmetic results with decreased blood loss and enhanced graft survival since the introduction of fibrin glue in burn care.[33]

Since the introduction of fibrin glue in our unit, debridement and resurfacing of facial aesthetic units with sheet grafts are done in a single procedure. Minimal blood loss and excellent graft stabilization associated with short and inexpensive postoperative care make this method attractive to patients and nursing personnel. Color and texture matches have been very satisfactory (Figs. 11-14 through 11-16).

A B C

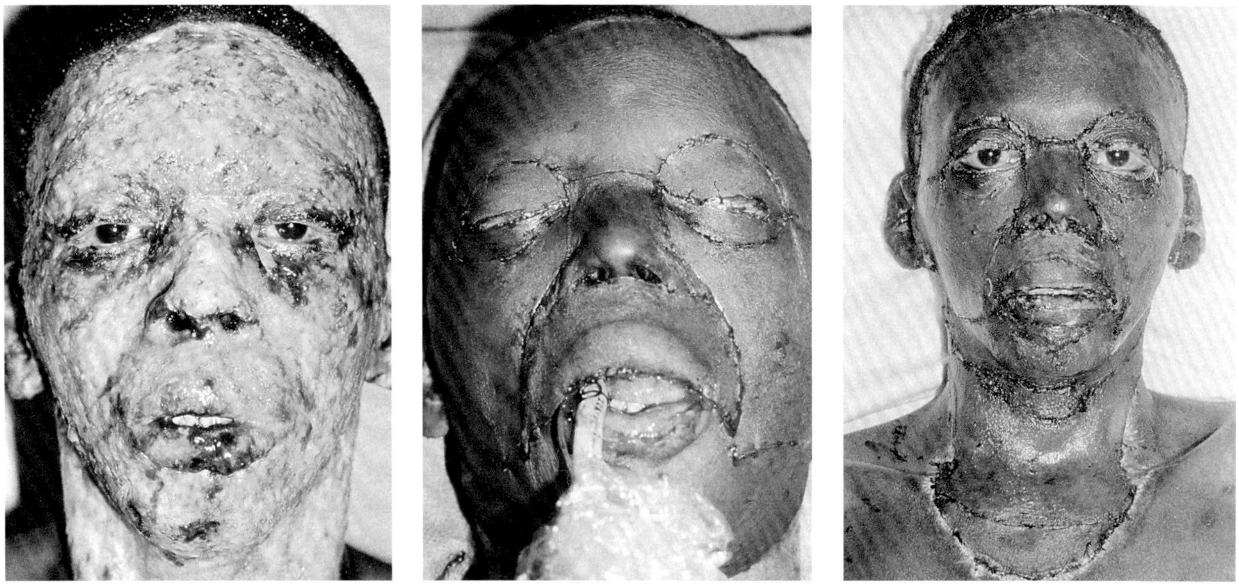

Figure 11-14 **A,** Ten days after facial burns; preoperative view. **B,** Debridement with immediate grafting of the aesthetic units of the face. **C,** Postoperative day 1. The patient was ambulatory without any dressings. (From Saltz R, Dimick A, Harris C, Grotting JC, Psillakis J, Vasconez LO. Application of autologous fibrin glue in burn wounds. J Burn Care Rehabil 10:504-507, 1989.)

A B

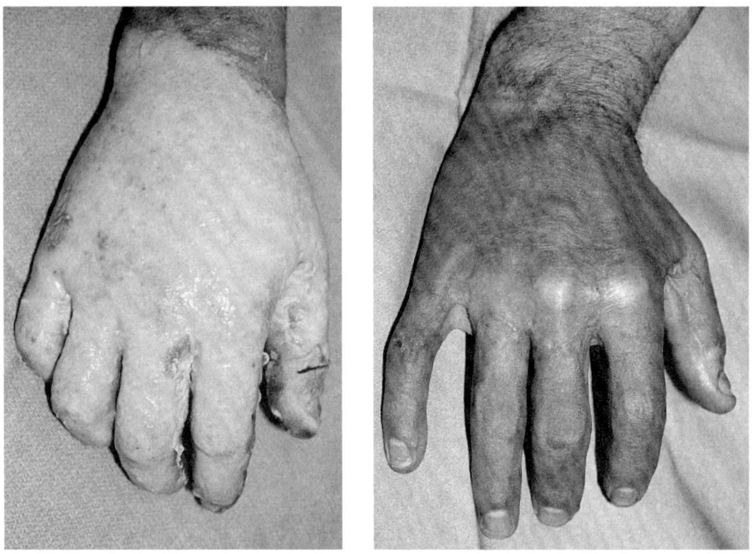

Figure 11-15 **A,** Deep partial-thickness burns of the hands. Active and passive motion exercise was started on postoperative day 2. **B,** At 5-month follow-up, the patient has full range of motion and an excellent aesthetic result. (**B,** From Saltz R, Sierra D, Feldman D, Saltz MB, Dimick A, Vasconez LO. Experimental and clinical applications of fibrin glue. Plast Reconstr Surg 88:1005-1015, 1991.)

A

B

C

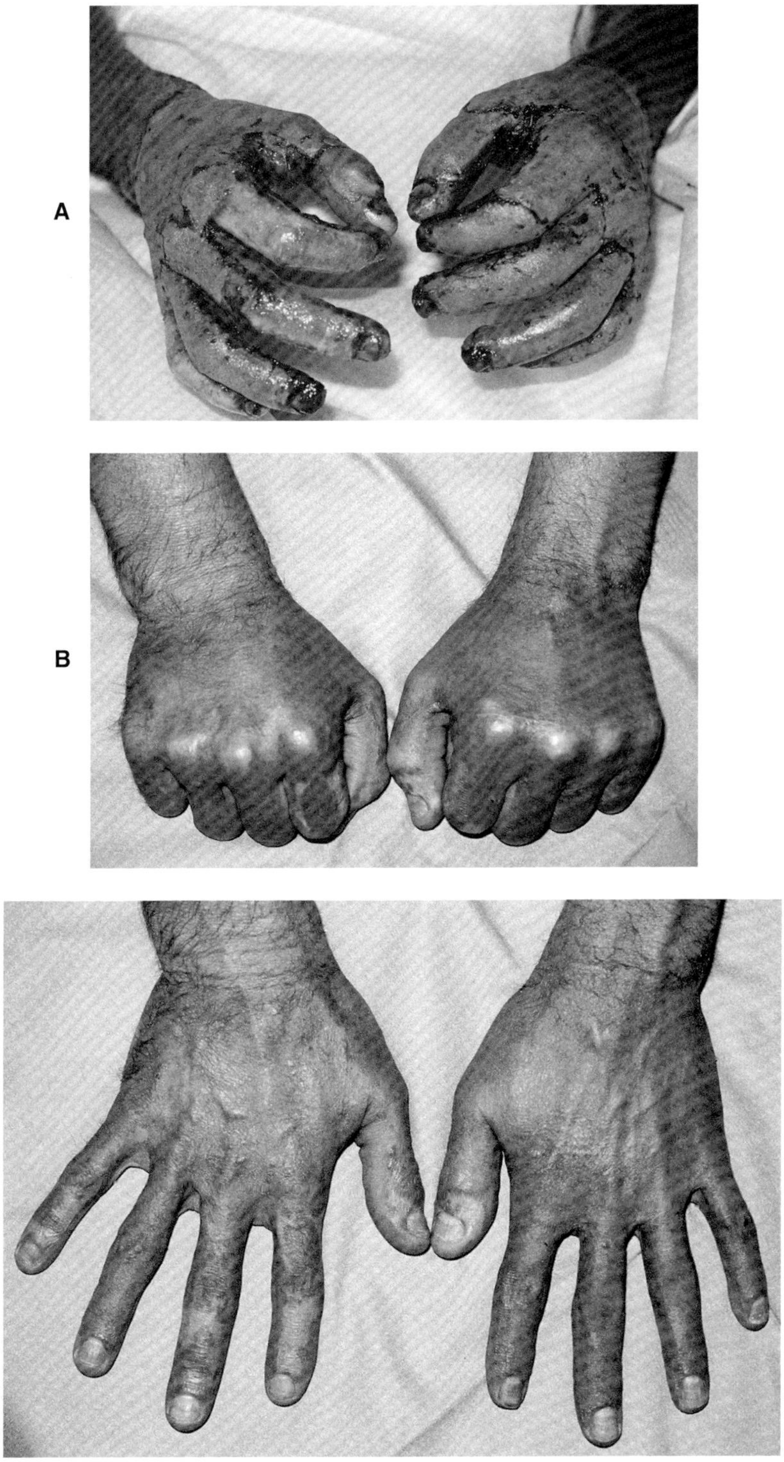

Figure 11-16 **A,** Four days after reconstruction of bilateral second- and third-degree burns of the hands. Split-thickness skin grafts secured with tissue glues allow early range of motion with no splints and no graft loss. **B** and **C,** Patient has full range of motion and excellent aesthetic results. (**A,** From Saltz R, Sierra D, Feldman D, Saltz MB, Dimick A, Vasconez LO. Experimental and clinical applications of fibrin glue. Plast Reconstr Surg 88:1005-1015, 1991.)

Future Directions

Throughout the centuries, surgeons and scientists have sought an ideal surgical sealant and adhesive, one that would be safe, biologically compatible, with rapid action and adequate tensile strength. In 1100 BC, Egyptians developed a variety of adhesives, using gum from acacia trees and several types of resin. Embalmed wounds were usually not sutured but sometimes were covered with a plate of beeswax. Surgical sutures have a well-established place in medicine. However, a variety of problems are encountered, including soft tissue incompatibility, which may result in fistulas or granulomas, absorbable material that may disintegrate early and cause dehiscence of the wound, and closely spaced sutures that may cause tissue ischemia, with resultant tissue necrosis of the wound margins. Cyanoacrylate-based substances, which were commonly used, are toxic to the tissues and can cause fistulization, granulomas, abscesses, and foreign body reaction. To overcome these problems, scientists continue their search for an adhesive that will ensure a perfect tissue union.

Currently used tissue glues represent significant advances over the adhesives first introduced in 1907. Efforts to improve tissue glues and expand applications are ongoing. The goal is an ideal adhesive that exhibits a number of properties conducive to wound healing. It should be able to bond tissue in place long enough to enable it to adhere without support. It should encourage tissue regeneration, support vascularization, and break down without any foreign body residue. Furthermore, it should be safe and not interfere with healing.

A number of new products and applications are currently under development. Some companies are working on products that apply tissue glues to wound dressings. These dressings could prove effective in the control of wounds that occur in battle because they would be applied directly to wounds to control local bleeding until they could be managed appropriately. Another application would be using a hemostatic tissue adhesive dressing in the operating room. These dressings would be applied directly over the wounds to control hemostasis and provide tissue adhesion. A third and promising dressing would be developed for use on burn patients.[14] These dressings would be bacteriostatic and moist enough to maintain the tissue viability. The dressings could be changed less frequently and possibly decrease the hospital stay for burn patients.

There is great potential for fibrin glue with skin grafts and tissue-engineered skin. Currie et al.[2] performed extensive research on the advantages and disadvantages of its use. Fibrin glue used with a reduced number of sutures may reduce thrombosis, stenosis, and vessel damage when combined with a telescoping technique of vessel repair. If used as a delivery system for cultured keratinocytes and fibroblasts, it may provide similar advantages to those associated with conventional skin grafts. So why not use it for all skin grafts? Currie et al.[2] noted that there is a risk of infection or reaction when blood products are being used, and the cost is significant. Storage and preparation time also have to be calculated in the decision to use a fibrin glue. Thus one must weigh the benefits and risks before using these products.

Some additional experimental applications of fibrin glue are to use it to adhere native cartilage to chondrocytes or tissue-engineered cartilage to fabricate cartilage constructs. Fibrin glue will become an important part of tissue-engineered skin replacements, and the use of exogenous growth factors may be a significant factor in accelerating wound healing.

Clinical and experimental research clearly demonstrates the potential for wide applicability of tissue glues as surgical and hemostatic agents. Although not a substitute for good surgical technique, the use of and applications for these adhesives should continue to grow as surgeons learn more about their capabilities. Decreased operating times and shorter hospital stays will have a positive impact on the economics and efficiency of plastic surgery practice, with substantial benefits to the patient and the surgeon.

REFERENCES

1. Jackson MR. Fibrin sealants in surgical practice: An overview. Am J Surg 182(2 Suppl):1S-7S, 2001.
2. Currie LJ, Sharpe JR, Martin R. The use of fibrin glue in skin grafts and tissue-engineered skin replacements: A review. Plast Reconstr Surg 108:1713-1726, 2001.
3. Rothenberg DM, Moy JN. Anaphylactic reaction to bovine thrombin anesthesiology. Anesthesiology 78:779-782, 1993.
4. Spotnitz WD, Dalton MS, Baker JW, Nolan SP. Successful use of fibrin glue during 2 years of surgery at a university medical center. Am Surg 55:166-168, 1989.
5. Staindl O. Tissue adhesion with highly concentrated fibrinogen in otolaryngology. Ann Otol Rhinol Laryngol 88:413-418, 1979.
6. Saltz R, Sierra D, Feldman D, Saltz MB, Dimick A, Vasconez LO. Experimental and clinical applications in fibrin glue. Plast Reconstr Surg 88:1005-1015, 1991.
7. Bruck HG. Fibrin glue tissue adhesion and its use in rhytidectomy: A pilot study. Aesthet Plast Surg 6:197-202, 1982.
8. Fezza JP, Cartwright M, Mack W, Flaharty P. The use of aerosolized fibrin glue in face lift surgery. Plast Reconstr Surg 110:658-664, 2002.
9. Marchac D, Sandor G. Facelifts and sprayed fibrin glue: An outcome analysis of 200 patients. Br J Plast Surg 47:306-309, 1994.
10. Trott AT. Cyanoacrylate tissue adhesives: An advance in wound care. JAMA 277:1559-1560, 1997.
11. Herod EL. Cyanoacrylates in dentistry: A review of the literature. J Can Dent Assoc 56:331-334, 1990.
12. Toriumi DM, O'Grady K, Desai D, Bagal A. Use of octyl-2-cyanoacrylate for skin closure in facial plastic surgery. Plast Reconstr Surg 102:2209-2219, 1998.
13. Wain J, Kaiser L, Johnstone D, Yang SC, Wright CD, Friedberg JS, Feins RH, Heitmiller RF, Mathisen DJ, Selwyn MR. Trial of a novel synthetic sealant in preventing air leaks after lung resection. Ann Thorac Surg 71:1628-1629, 2001.
14. Reece TB, Maxey TS, Kron IL. A prospectus on tissue adhesives. Am J Surg 182(2 Suppl): 40S-44S, 2001.

15. Oz MC, Cosgrove DM III, Badduke BR, Hill JD, Flannery MR, Palumbo R, Topic N. Controlled clinical trial of a novel hemostatic agent in cardiac surgery. The Fusion Matrix Study Group. Ann Thorac Surg 69:1376-1382, 2001.
16. Renkens KL Jr, Payner TD, Leipzig TJ, Feuer H, Morone MA, Koers JM, Lawson KJ, Lentz R, Shuey H Jr, Conaway GL, Andersson GB, An HS, Hickey M, Rondinone JF, Shargill NS. A multicenter, prospective, randomized trial evaluating a new hemostatic agent for spinal surgery. Spine 26:1645-1650, 2001.
17. Grossman JA, Capraro PA, Burneikis V. Minimizing complications in the use of fibrin sealant in aesthetic facial procedures. Aesthet Surg J 21:32-39, 2001.
18. Vibe P, Pless J. A new method of skin graft adhesion. Scand J Plast Reconstr Surg 17:263-264, 1983.
19. Greenhalgh DG, Gamelli RL, Lee M, Delavari M, Lynch JB, Hansbrough JF, Achauer BM, Miller SF, MacPhee M, Bray GL. Multicenter trial to evaluate the safety and potential efficacy of pooled human fibrin sealant for the treatment of burn wounds. J Trauma 46:433-440, 1999.
20. Adant JPH, Detroz B, Natowitz SL, Ledoue M, Pestau B, LeClerq D. Skin grafting with fibrin glue in burns. Eur J Plast Surg 16:292-297, 1993.
21. Chakravorty RC, Sosnowski K. Autologous fibrin glue in full thickness skin grafting. Ann Plast Surg 23:488-491, 1989.
22. Gosain AK, Lyon VB. The current status of tissue glues: Part II. For adhesion of soft tissues (safety and efficacy report). Plast Reconstr Surg 110:1581-1584, 2002.
23. Spotnitz WD, Dalton MS, Baker JW, Noan SP. Successful use of fibrin glue during 2 years of surgery at a university medical center. Am Surg 55:166-168, 1989.
24. Ihara N, Suzuki K, Tanaka H. Application of fibrin glue to burns: Its haemostatic and skin transplant fixation effects in the excised wound. Burns Incl Therm Inj 10:396-404, 1984.
25. Stuart JD, Kenney JG, Lettieri J, Spotnitz W, Baker J. Application of single-donor fibrin glue to burns. J Burn Care Rehabil 9:619-622, 1988.
26. Ellis DA, Pelausa EO. Fibrin glues in facial plastic and reconstructive surgery. J Otolaryngol 17:74-77, 1988.
27. Moro H, Hayashi J, Ohzeki H, Hakayama T, Namura O, Hanzawa K, Yagi N. The effect of fibrin glue on inhibition of pericardial adhesions. Thorac Cardiovasc Surg 47:79-84, 1999.
28. Toosie K, Callego K, Stabile BE, Schaber B, French S, de Virgilio C. Fibrin glue reduces intra-abdominal adhesions to synthetic mesh in a rat ventral hernia model. Am Surg 66:41-45, 2000.
29. Arnold PB, Green CW, Foresman PA, Rodeheaver GT. Evaluation of resorbable barriers for preventing surgical adhesions. Fertil Steril 73:157-161, 2000.
30. Meek K, de Virgilio C, Murell Z, Karamatsu M, Stabile B, Amin S, Sandoval M, French S, Pierre K. Inhibition of intra-abdominal adhesions: A comparison of Hemaseel APR and cryoprecipitate fibrin glue. J Invest Surg 14:227-233, 2001.
31. Kulber DA, Bacilious N, Peters ED, Gayle LB, Hoffman L. The use of fibrin sealant in the prevention of seromas. Plast Reconstr Surg 99:842-849; discussion 850-851, 1997.
32. Gibble JW, Ness PM. Fibrin glue: The perfect operative sealant? Transfusion 30:741-747, 1990.
33. Saltz R, Dimick A, Harris C, Grottin JC, Psillakis J, Vasconez LO. Application of autologous fibrin glue in burn wounds. J Burn Care Rehabil 10:504-507, 1989.
34. Saltz R, Sierra D, Feldman D, Bartczak Saltz M, Dimick A, Vasconez LO. Experimental and clinical applications of fibrin glue. Plast Reconstr Surg 88:1005-1015, 1991.
35. Janzekovic Z. A new concept in the early excision and immediate grafting of burns. J Trauma 10:1103-1108, 1970.
36. Engrav LH, Hembach DM, Walkinshaw MD, Marvin JA. Excision of burns of the face. Plast Reconstr Surg 77:744-751, 1986.
37. Casagrande C, Saltz R, Chem R, Pinto R, Collares M. Direct needle fixation in endoscopic facial rejuvenation. Aesthetic Surg J 20:361-367, 2000.

INDEX

MARKETING AGRICULTURAL COMMODITIES

Farm Business Management

FBM14101NC

Marketing and price risk management
in agricultural commodities.

John Deere